Clinical Cases in Ophthalmology

Erratum Slip for Clinical Cases in Ophthalmology (Hoh and Easty)

Case	Page/Line	Correction
Case 1.6	12/1	Four should read twelve.
Case 1.9	16/2	There is a word missing from this sentence. It should read: The cornea is **clear** above and below and has a clear margin at the limbus.
Case 2.1	36/4	FFA should read anterior segment fluorescein angiogram.
	36/11	The drug oxyphenbutazone has been withdrawn from the market.
Case 3.7	65/4	Epidermal should read epibulbar.
Case 3.11	72/18	*Streptococcus* should read *Staphylococcus*.
Case 3.15	80/1	There are several words missing from this sentence. It should read: Active inflammation **involving the posterior segment can** be treated with immunosupression such as steroids or steroid-sparing agents such as cyclosporin and azathioprine.
Case 5.2	105/2	Superotemporal should read inferotemporal.
Case 5.12	125/11	Haematoma should read hamartoma.
Case 6.4	151/2	Cotton wool spots with no loss should read cotton wool spots with **complete** loss.
Case 8.1	175/25	AZT should read Azathioprine.
Case 8.5	182/1	Ptosis in the right eye should read ptosis in the left eye.
Case 8.12	197/30	Ophthalmic stripping should read: Excision of the eyelid protractors combined with a brow lift (Anderson's procedure).

Clinical Cases in
Ophthalmology

H.B. Hoh FRCOphth

D.L. Easty MD FRCS FRCOphth

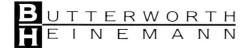

Butterworth-Heinemann Ltd
Linacre House, Jordan Hill, Oxford OX2 8DP

℞ A member of the Reed Elsevier group

OXFORD LONDON BOSTON
MUNICH NEW DELHI SINGAPORE SYDNEY
TOKYO TORONTO WELLINGTON

First published 1995

British Library Cataloguing in Publication Data
Hoh, H. B.
    Clinical Cases in Ophthalmology
    I. Title II. Easty, David L.
    617.7

ISBN 0 7506 2102 8

Library of Congress Cataloguing in Publication Data
Hoh, H. B.
    Clinical cases in ophthalmology/H.B. Hoh, D.L. Easty.
    p.   cm.
    Includes bibliographical references and index.
    ISBN 0 7506 2102 8
    1. Ophthalmology--Case studies. 2. Eye--Diseases--Case studies.
    I. Easty, D. L. II. Title.
    [DNLM: 1. Eye Diseases – diagnosis – case studies. 2. Eye Diseases –
    therapy – case studies. WW 140 H717c 1995]
    RE69.H64 1995   94-44574
    617.7'1–dc20   CIP

Composition by Scribe Design, Gillingham, Kent
Printed in Spain

Contents

Preface

Final specialist examination has become more difficult as the competition to train as an ophthalmologist increases. Most candidates find difficulty at the vivas and clinical examination where they can be shown slides or patients with signs that may not be familiar. This is especially true when candidates have not had an opportunity to work at a referral centre incorporating specialities such as orbital, oculoplastics or vitreoretinal units.

Clinical Cases in Ophthalmology is written to provide examples of the sort of challenging cases that may be presented to a candidate. It is designed not so much as a text of didactic teaching but one that helps the candidate to point out the main positive *and* negative signs that should be elicited and how to present a suitable list of differential diagnoses. Examiners will judge the candidates according to their competence in demonstrating relevant signs and their management of the patient. The candidate is encouraged to discuss the management based on the signs seen and *not* word for word parrot-fashion out of a textbook. Instead, the candidate should point out the indications for intervention and the various therapeutic options that are currently available.

Where possible, the prognosis of the condition is stated. There are often 'tips' given such as looking for bilaterality of a condition or evidence of previous surgery. Finally a number of key articles is cited to encourage the candidate to be as up-to-date as possible as textbooks become dated rather quickly in the rapidly expanding field of ophthalmology.

We would like to wish all candidates the best of luck!

H.B.H.
D.L.E.

How to use this book

The book contains 100 clinical cases divided into eight sections according to the anatomy. They are chosen to be challenging and to encourage the reader to think and read around the subject. In this way, the book aims to cover as much ophthalmology as possible and to ensure that the reader has a clear and methodical approach to solving each problem. There is an illustration of a clinical case (or in some cases a Hess chart or fluorescein angiogram) presented with clear signs on each page. We have chosen not to give any clues by providing a case history as this will defeat the object of the exercise. The reader is encouraged to pick out the signs and make sense of the case by discussing it (see Clinical examination technique).

The discussion of each case appears on the page overleaf and is laid out as follows.

1. Description of the slide consisting of
    - positive signs
    - relevant negative findings
    - differential diagnosis and most likely diagnosis.
2. Investigations.
3. Management, which follows the order of
    - conservative
    - medical
    - laser
    - surgical.
4. Prognosis and relevant information of the disorder.
5. Top tips.

Using this pedantic method of examination, the candidate is unlikely to miss subtle signs. It is hoped that this approach will be used when practising in mock situations so that in the presence of the examiners, little will go amiss.

Clinical examination technique

At the clinical examination, patients with clinical signs will be presented to the candidate along with relevant Hess charts, fluorescein angiograms or visual fields. Although the examiner may provide some background history to the case, most will say little and proceed to present the patient to you. The examiner will instruct you to examine the relevant anatomy of the eye or orbit. You are then on your own.

1. 'Have a look at the cornea/anterior segment/macula/fundus/disc and tell us what you see' usually starts the examination. This is your cue to look at the relevant part of the eye and comment on the signs seen beginning with the most obvious. (Note: do not waste time describing normal findings.) Then comment on any relevant negative findings; these are signs which may be associated with the diagnosis but are absent in the case presented to you or signs which help rule out other differential diagnosis. Finally you should provide a list of the diagnoses to the examiner, pick the most suitable one to fit your case and explain your choice. Begin with the commonest causes first and leave rare differential diagnosis to the end.

Take for example Case 3.9, the iris melanoma. The examiner will ask you to look at the anterior segment. You should begin by describing the obvious iris lesion by its size, shape, position, colour, pigmentation, extrascleral extension etc. Then look for relevant negative findings; in this case mention the absence of raised intraocular pressure, cataract or subluxation of the lens which may be caused by the lesion. By this time you should have the differential diagnosis of iris lesions at hand. Iris melanoma will be at the top of the list as it fits the description you have given. You should also then suggest other lesions such as a naevus or neurofibroma which may look like it.

2. This may lead the examiner to ask how you would investigate the case to differentiate the various lesions you have suggested. As with any clinical cases seen in clinical practice, only the minimum and relevant investigations should be used to elucidate the correct diagnosis. This is the basis of competent and sound clinical practice. Relevant ocular, systemic and family history should be taken before embarking on more sophisticated tests. The candidate should be familiar with the principles of the techniques used and their interpretation. It would be foolish to perform, say, a fluorescein angiogram when the clinician does not know what to expect. As such, do not be surprised when asked to describe the positive features you would expect to see to confirm your diagnosis in any of the investigations you have listed.

3.   Having confirmed the diagnosis (hopefully the correct one), it is obvious that you will need to know what to do and when to do it. Do not forget that there are times when observation is the prudent management of choice. For example, inactive toxoplasmosis scar (Case 5.6) does not require intervention unless the lesion becomes active. Even then, there are strict criteria as the systemic treatment is potentially toxic and should only be given when indicated.

In some cases, there may be a choice of treatment. For example, there are medical, laser and surgical treatments available for the treatment of open angle glaucoma (Case 3.4). As such you should be able to describe the various options available and discuss why or when one may be more suitable than the other. You should have knowledge of the technique, side-effects, complications and outcome of the treatment modalities. Do not forget that even if the condition is beyond treatment and the vision irreversibly damaged, the patient can be offered low-visual aids and rehabilitation.

4.   Finally, it is good practice to inform on the prognosis of the condition and the expected visual outcome. In the case of chronic conditions such as age-related macular degeneration, the patient should be informed of the small but definite risk of a subretinal neovascular membrane which manifests as metamorphopsia. An Amsler chart could be issued to the patient prior to discharge from the clinician's care.

In the examination, you should manage the case presented as you would usually manage it in the outpatient clinic. Do not panic if you come across an unfamiliar case but continue to run through the signs logically as described above. It may turn out to be a case of unknown aetiology with no correct answer but the examiners will be judging you on your approach in handling the case in a sensible manner. Remember that examiners are *not* out to fail you but to ensure that candidates are competent and safe in the management of both straightforward and more complex cases.

Equipment required for clinical examination

It is important to be equipped with the appropriate instruments and diagnostic tools that you are familiar with in the examination. It is always prudent to bring your own instruments. Nothing can be more unnerving than to fumble around with an instrument that has run out of batteries or is unfamiliar to you! In preparation for the examination, see patients in 'full battle dress'; i.e. complete with the same pieces of equipment that you will be bringing to the examination. This will enable you to know precisely which coat pocket houses your 90D lens, and where you have placed your red pin.

The examiners can easily tell whether you have performed a cover–uncover test or tested pupillary reflexes the moment you approach the patient. When you have performed a test for long enough, all your actions are automatic; there should be no hesitant gaps as you think what to do next. We strongly recommend that you not only practise regularly but perform the examination in the correct manner. Do not take short cuts! Your bad habits will manifest in front of the examiners.

We recommend that the following should be at hand in the examination:

1. A 90 or 78 dioptres lens for visualizing the macula on the slit-lamp.
2. A 20 dioptres lens for visualizing the fundus with the indirect ophthalmoscope.
3. An ophthalmoscope with new batteries (usually for disc visualization or red reflexes).
4. Pen torch to examine the pupillary reflexes.
5. A red (or white pin) to
   - examine blind spots and visual fields on confrontation
   - detect red desaturation secondary to an optic nerve lesion.
6. An occluder to perform cover–uncover test in strabismus.
7. A fixation target for a child (toy) and an adult (reduced Snellen print) to
   - perform cover–uncover test for near
   - elicit pupil constriction on near gaze
   - demonstrate extraocular movements in the cardinal positions of gaze.
8. A ruler (in metric scale) to measure the size of
   - a skin lesion
   - a ptosis
   - a proptosis
   - the pupils.

Cornea

Graft rejection

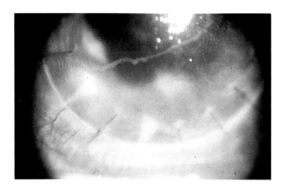

There is a horizontal line of keratic precipitates on the endothelium (Khodadoust line) of a penetrating keratoplasty which is slightly oedematous and containing inflammatory infiltrates. This is suggestive of an acute corneal host-versus-graft rejection. Other signs include Krachmer spots, deep and superficial vascularization and anterior uveitis. Risk factors contributing to corneal graft rejection are pre-existing corneal vascularization and re-grafts.[1] Rejections occur in 1–5% of penetrating keratoplasties.

Pathologically, graft rejection is a combination of type 1 and 4 hypersensitivity reaction. It is due to the recognition of the MHC type 2 antigens of Langerhans cells present in the donor cornea by host T-lymphocytes at the graft–host interface. The presence of corneal vascularization increases such a risk.

Investigations

(a)   Herpes simplex titres to exclude disciform keratitis.
(b)   Specular microscopy is useful at a later stage to assess extent of damage to endothelial cell density following the rejection episode.

Management

Treat early and aggressively to prevent unnecessary damage to the endothelium.

1.   Intensive topical steroids such as hourly dexamethasone to reduce the inflammatory response.
2.   Systemic immunosuppression using steroids, cyclosporin or azathioprine may be required if the inflammatory response is severe.[2]
3.   Patient should be warned of the symptoms of possible rejection episodes (blurred, uncomfortable red eye) for future reference. In high-risk grafts, the patients may require low-dose immunosuppression on a regular basis postoperatively.

4 Clinical cases in ophthalmology

Tips

Know the side-effects of all immunosuppressant therapy.

References

1. Wilson, S.E. and Kaufman, H.E. (1990) Graft failure after penetrating keratoplasty. *Survey of Ophthalmology*, **34**, 325–56
2. Hill, J.C. (1989) The use of cyclosporin in high-risk keratoplasty. *American Journal of Ophthalmology*, **107**, 506–10

Cytotoxic – Azathioprine

s/e myelosupp

hepatotoxicits

Immunosuppressant

alkylating

Cyclophosphamide

Keratoconjunctivitis sicca

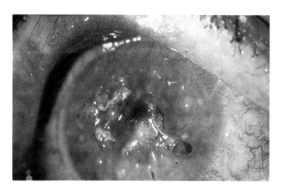

There are mucus filaments and punctate corneal epitheliopathy (or punctate erosions) in the inferior part of the cornea. Other signs include a poor tear film and mild hyperaemia. This is consistent with keratoconjunctivitis sicca (KCS) which has many causes:

- Idiopathic (age-related).
- Primary Sjögren's syndrome (autoimmune disease characterized by lymphocytic infiltration and destruction of the lacrimal and salivary glands resulting in KCS and xerostomia in the absence of any systemic disease).
- Secondary Sjögren's syndrome (KCS and xerostomia associated with systemic diseases such as rheumatoid arthritis, systemic lupus erythematosus, sarcoidosis, systemic sclerosis, Hashimoto's thyroiditis and primary biliary cirrhosis.
- Lacrimal infiltration with tumours (such as lymphoma) or infection (tuberculosis).
- Scarring and subsequent blockage of excretory ducts of the lacrimal gland due to a cicatricial process such as chemical burns, radiation to the orbit, pemphigoid or Stevens–Johnson syndrome.

Investigations

(a) Exclude any associated systemic disease.
(b) Measurement of the tear film break-up time (BUT) will assess the integrity of the corneal tear film.
(c) Staining of corneal epithelial defects with fluorescein.
(d) Staining of devitalized epithelial cells and mucus filaments with Rose Bengal 1%.
(e) Schirmer's test measures the tear production of the tear glands.
(f) Tear osmolality is increased in dry eye states.
(g) Conjunctiva imprint cytology or biopsy can estimate the conjunctival goblet cell density.

Management

Management is directed at maintaining the tear film, keeping the eye comfortable and preventing complications which may arise.

1.   Conservative measures
     • Goggles and humidifiers help to conserve tears.
2.   Medical treatment
     • Tear substitutes can be cellulose based (Hypromellose), polyvinyl based (Liquifilm) or mucomimetics (Tears Naturale).
     • Mucolytics such as acetylcysteine 5% (Ilube) remove excessive mucus.
3.   Surgery
     • Punctal occlusion using punctal plugs, diathermy or suture.
     • Tarsorrhaphy reduces the area of cornea exposed to drying.

Prognosis

There is no permanent cure for KCS.

Corneal granular dystrophy

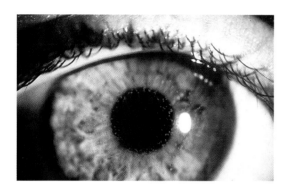

There are multiple discrete whitish corneal opacities scattered throughout the cornea but sparing the periphery. They are in the stromal layer and the cornea in between the opacities is clear. This is consistent with granular form (Groenouw type 1) which is one of several types of corneal stromal dystrophies (the others being lattice and macular).

Differential diagnosis

Includes Reis–Buckler's anterior corneal dystrophy, Schnyder central crystalline dystrophy and lattice stromal dystrophy.

Investigations

(a) The diagnosis is a clinical one.
(b) Examination of relatives will confirm the dominant inheritance of this condition.
(c) Histology of the specimen shows deposition of rod-shaped non-collagenous protein deposits which are electron dense on electron microscopy and stain bright red with Masson trichrome.

Management

Although the condition begins to manifest at the age of 10 years, the condition is usually asymptomatic until the third decade when vision may be disturbed by glare or rarely corneal erosions. No treatment is necessary until vision has deteriorated sufficiently to require a penetrating keratoplasty.

Prognosis

Opacities may recur in the graft at a later stage.

Case 1.4

Reis–Buckler's corneal dystrophy

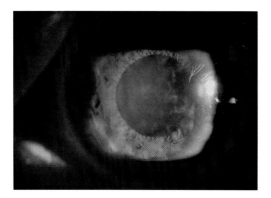

There are many ring-shaped opacities giving a 'honeycombed' appearance at the level of Bowman's membrane in the centre of the cornea which may extend to the periphery. This is consistent with a Reis–Buckler's anterior dystrophy which may cause epithelial problems leading to recurrent corneal erosions and visual disturbance due to light scatter.

Differential diagnosis

Includes anterior crocodile shageen patch. There are two variants to this condition:

- Anterior membrane dystrophy (Grayson–Hilbrant), which has a better prognosis as the cornea is relatively clear between the opacities, the peripheral cornea is spared and the vision less affected.
- Honeycombed dystrophy (Thiel and Behnke), which is associated with severe recurrent corneal erosions.

Investigations

(a) The diagnosis is a clinical one.
(b) Examination of relatives will confirm the dominant inheritance of this condition.
(c) Histology of the specimen shows degeneration of Bowman's membrane which in areas is replaced by scar tissue of variable thickness. The overlying epithelium may show degeneration which heralds the erosion process.

Management

Although in the early stages the patient may be asymptomatic, most patients will have problems of visual disturbance or recurrent erosions by the third decade. There are two surgical options:

1.   Lamellar keratoplasty.
2.   Penetrating keratoplasty.

Prognosis

Opacities may recur in the graft at a later stage.

Keratoconus

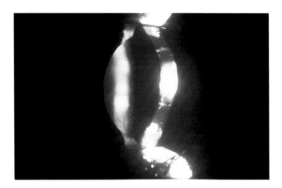

There is thinning and distortion of the cornea with a small central opacity. This is consistent with keratoconus, an ectatic dystrophy which is bilateral in nature and occurs in 1 in 20 000, especially in Down's syndrome, atopic patients, Marfan's syndrome, Ehlers–Danlos syndrome and osteogenesis imperfecta. Other features seen are fine vertical folds (Vogt's lines) which disappear on pressure to the eye, prominent corneal nerves, Fleischer's iron ring (best seen with cobalt light), slit-lamp light sharply focused on to nasal limbus (Rizzutti sign), bulging of the eyelid on looking down (Munson's sign) and central opacity complicated by a previous episode of hydrops.

Differential diagnosis

Includes keratoglobus.

Investigations

(a) Refraction (the 'oil-drop' sign can be seen with the retinoscope) and keratoscopy.
(b) Corneal topographical mapping using Placido's disc or a computed topographical system.

Management

The main problem with the ectasia is progressive irregular astigmatism of the cornea causing visual problems. The visual problem can be solved by:

1. Spectacles initially.
2. Contact lens.
3. Surgery either with epikeratophakia or penetrating keratoplasty when the patient becomes either contact lens intolerant or the astigmatism is no longer controlled by contact lenses.

Prognosis

Over 90% of the grafts for penetrating keratoplasty remain clear after 5 years and visual rehabilitation is excellent. There may be a problem with a dilated pupil postoperatively (Ureth–Zavalia phenomenon).

Radial keratotomy

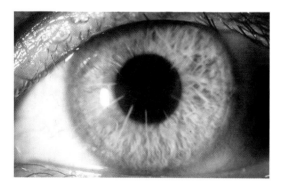

There are four deep radial incisions in the cornea with a clear 4 mm central portion. This is radial keratotomy, a form of refractive surgery for myopia.[1,2] Other surgical procedures for myopia include:

- Excimer laser.
- Keratomieliusis.
- Epikeratophakia.

Management

The patient should be warned of the complications of radial keratotomy which are microperforations, bacterial keratitis, glare, recurrent erosions, weakening of the cornea at the incisions and return of the original myopia. Diurnal fluctuation of vision is also a common complaint.

Prognosis[3]

At 3 years postoperatively, 76% of eyes had an unaided visual acuity of 6/12 or better. The major factors affecting the change in refraction were the diameter of the clear optical zone, the depth of the incision scar and the number of incisions.

References

1. Forstot, S.L. (1988) Radial keratotomy. *International Ophthalmic Clinics*, **28**, 116–25
2. American Academy of Ophthalmology (1993). Radial keratotomy for myopia. *Ophthalmology*, **100**, 1103–15
3. Waring, G.O., Lynn, M.J., and Culbertson, W. (1987) Three-year results of the Prospective Evaluation of Radial Keratotomy (PERK) Study. *Ophthalmology*, **94**, 1339–54

Pseudophakic bullous keratopathy

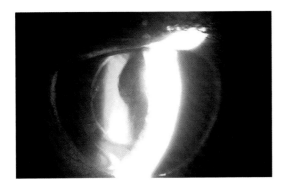

There is diffuse corneal oedema throughout all layers of the cornea in an otherwise non-inflamed pseudophakic eye. There appears to be an anterior chamber intraocular lens. This is an example of endothelial decompensation due to either chronic raised intraocular pressure or secondary to the presence of the anterior intraocular lens. Pseudophakic bullous keratopathy is the commonest indication for corneal graft.[1]

Differential diagnosis

Includes:

- Low endothelial density due to excessive endothelial loss during the original procedure (there is an estimated 10–15% loss of endothelium in a cataract procedure) or trauma.
- Endothelial dystrophy such as Fuch's endothelial dystrophy (more likely to be bilateral with evidence of guttatae), posterior polymorphous dystrophy or irido-corneal endothelial syndrome.
- Co-existing glaucoma.
- Previous chronic intraocular inflammation.

Investigations

(a) A specular microscopic assessment of the endothelial cell count of both eyes to exclude a bilateral condition such as Fuch's dystrophy.
(b) The intraocular pressure should be measured to exclude glaucoma as a cause.

Management

Management may involve doing nothing if the patient is able to function with the fellow eye in the early stage and does not want surgical intervention. However, the patient is likely to suffer pain from epithelial oedema, haloes and loss of vision as the oedema progresses. The treatment options are:

1. Medical treatment includes hyperosmotic agents such as 5% saline or glycerol when needed. A hairdryer over the face can aid evaporation and reduce oedema especially on waking. Soft bandage contact lens protects the cornea and keeps the eye comfortable.
2. Surgical treatment involves a penetrating keratoplasty, ideally with a fresh donor with high endothelial cell density. Removal of the anterior intraocular lens is difficult but important to prevent recurrence. The option of replacing the implant with a posterior chamber implant is debatable as it would need either scleral fixation or iris fixation which could be technically awkward. However, leaving the patient aphakic in one eye may cause aniesokonia unless the patient is able to tolerate a contact lens.

Reference

1. Speaker, M.G., Lugo M., and Liabson, P.R. (1988) Penetrating keratoplasty for pseudophakic bullous keratopathy. *Ophthalmology*, **95**, 1260–8

Case 1.8

Postoperative astigmatism

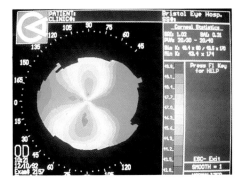

This is a computed topographical picture of an eye with asymmetrical astigmatism with steepness at axis 90° suggestive of a postoperative cataract or trabeculectomy or with-the-rule astigmatism. Computed topography uses the principles of Placido's disc and maps out lines of isodioptres. These are colour coded with red for steep areas and blue for flat areas.

Management

Management of postoperative astigmatism is important to prevent aniseikonia.

1. *Early postoperative period* When sutures are still in place these can be selectively removed at the axis of steepness (i.e. tight sutures) at a reasonable period postoperatively when the wound has healed sufficiently and would not dehiesce.
2. *Late* When a patient presents late, when there are no longer any sutures remaining, then the options are:[1]
   • Contact lens if the astigmatism is small.
   • Relaxing keratotomy (at the steep areas) or/and compression sutures (at the flat areas).
   • Excimer laser with variable aperture.

Reference

1. Kaufman, H.E., McDonald, M.B., Barron, B.A. and Wilson, S.E. (1992) *Colour Atlas of Ophthalmic Surgery. Corneal and Refractive Surgery.* J.B. Lippincott, Philadelphia, pp. 309–30

Corneal band keratopathy

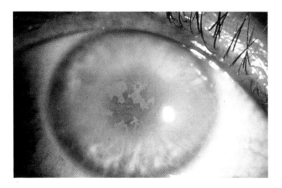

There is a horizontal band of opacity at the subepithelial level at the inter-palpebral region. The cornea is above and below and has a clear margin at the limbus. Deposition of calcium plaques with 'holes' can be seen throughout the band. This is consistent with band keratopathy which is associated with:

- Idiopathic origin.
- Ocular causes such as chronic iridocyclitis in juvenile chronic arthritis, phthsis bulbi, chronic exposure and repeated corneal trauma.
- Systemic hypercalcaemic states.

Differential diagnosis

Includes lipid keratopathy, amyloid degeneration (gelatinous drop-like dystrophy of the cornea) and Salzmann's nodular dystrophy.

Investigations

(a) Unnecessary due to obvious clinical diagnosis.
(b) If necessary, a corneal biopsy will reveal calcium deposition in the plane between the epithelium and Bowman's membrane.

Management

The underlying problem should be rectified first although such cases usually present late.

1. *Early* In the early stages, the lesion is often asymptomatic and no treatment may be required.
2. *Late* An advanced band often causes dry eye symptoms due to disruption of the tear film or pain if there is epithelium erosion. Vision is affected when the band encroaches on the visual axis. Treatment is aimed at the removal of the band and the options are:

- Scraping with a knife.
- Calcium chelating agents such as sodium versenate or disodium ethylenediamine tetra-acetic acid (EDTA).
- Excimer laser.

Acanthamoeba keratitis

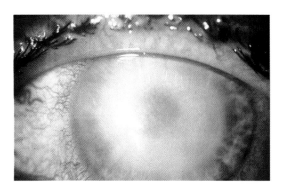

There is a round area of infiltrate in the centre of the cornea in a hyper-aemic eye. There is no evidence of anterior chamber activity or hypopyon and this may suggest an infective keratitis such as Acanthamoeba, bacterial, herpes simplex virus or fungal origin. The symptoms of photophobia and unusually extreme pain are suggestive of Acanthamoeba keratitis. Other features include central ring-shaped infiltrates, epithelial defects, scleritis and pathoneumonic stromal opacities extending inwards from the limbus in a radial manner along the corneal nerves called perineural infiltrates or radial keratoneuritis.

In addition, a history of trauma, contact lens wear or contamination with soil, points towards an infective cause due to Acanthamoeba.

Investigations

Investigations revolve around the identification of the organism through microscopy, staining (Gram, Giemsa, Gomori's silver stain), immunofluorescent antibody techniques and culture (on an agar plate with confluent growth of *E. coli* bacteria) of the sample derived from:

(a) Swabbing of the surface ocular structures like the conjunctiva.
(b) Scrape of the corneal infiltrate.
(c) Culture of contact lens and lens solution if appropriate.

Management

The principle relies on prompt diagnosis, and treatment is aimed at eradicating the two forms of this protozoa – the dormant cysts and the motile trophozoites. This takes the form of:

1. Combination therapy of topical propamidine isethionate 0.1% and polyhexamethylene biguanide on an hourly basis.[1] Neomycin should also be given concurrently.

2. Analgesia such as oral flurbiprofen 500 mg three times daily for the pain.
3. Weak topical steroids reduce inflammation but should be used with caution.[2]
4. Therapeutic penetrating keratoplasty to reduce infective organism load is indicated when there is persistent inflammation and pain despite medical treatment, or impending corneal perforation.

Prognosis

Final outcomes can be 6/12 or better in 80% of cases.[3] Polymicrobial keratitis should be suspected if there is a poor response to treatment or if new infiltrates begin to appear.

References

1. Larkin, D.F.P., Kilvington, S. and Dart, J.K.G. (1992) Treatment of Acanthamoeba keratitis with polyhexamethylene biguanide. *Ophthalmology*, **99**, 185–91
2. Stern, G.A., and Buttross, M. (1991) Use of corticosteroids in combination with antimicrobial drugs in the treatment of infectious corneal disease. *Ophthalmology*, **98**; 847-853
3. Bacon, A.S., Frazer, D.G., Dart, J.K.G. (1993) A review of 72 consecutive cases of Acanthamoeba keratitis, 1982–1992. *Eye*, **7**, 719–25

Donor corneal–scleral disc

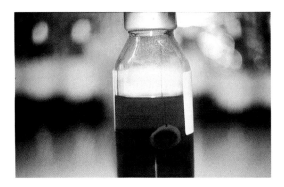

This is a corneal–scleral disc suspended in pink organ medium culture which is used for corneal grafting (either penetrating or lamellar keratoplasty). This method of corneal storage is called the **organ culture** technique and offers the following advantages:

- Regularize supply to meet demand thus preventing wastage.
- Planning of elective surgery.
- Donor screening of HIV, Hep B/C and bacterial infection.
- Donor quality assessment (e.g. quantifying endothelial cell density).
- Tissue typing in high risk patients.

The following are types of corneal storage currently in use.

1. **Moist chamber at 4°C**, which involves hypothermic storage of whole eyes and needs to be used within 48 hours.

2. **Hypothermic storage of corneal-scleral disc in organ culture at 4°C**, popularised by McCarey and Kaufman since 1974 in the USA. The culture medium (originally containing 5% dextran and gentamycin, and named after them as the M–K medium) consists of 5% dextran, Hepes buffer and antibiotics (penicillin and streptomycin). This method allows corneal clarity for up to 7 days.

3. **Cryopresevation**. The discovery of glycerol in 1949 and later dimethyl sulphoxide as cryopreservants has led to successful cryopreservation of many biological materials. This is due to the stability of tissues at –196°C (boiling point of liquid nitrogen) as no chemical reactions can occur below –130°C. Although successful grafts have been achieved, the donor tissues were chosen to be optimal (age less than 50 years and were processed within 6 hours). The problem with freezing is that there is formation of intracellular ice which can cause up to 70% cell loss within 1 year of grafting.

4. **Organ culture at 37°C**, described by Doughman and Lindstrom in 1976. Organ culture has been shown to have similar success rates

postoperatively (80% of grafts were clear) as the previous methods. During culture, the cornea swells to about twice the normal thickness but by placing the cornea in culture medium containing 5% w/v dextran the cornea returns to its previous size within 12–24 hours. This method allows storage of corneas for up 28 days and accounts for over 80% of all corneas used for corneal grafts in the United Kingdom.

Corneal verticillata (of Fleischer)

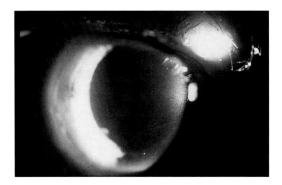

There are golden-grey epithelial deposits which originate from the centre (more correctly referred to as epicentre) towards the periphery in a vortex pattern. This is a bilateral condition called vortex keratopathy (or corneal verticillata).

Differential diagnosis

Includes systemic treatment with drugs such as amiodarone, chloroquine, chlorpromazine and tamoxifen. It is also found in Fabry's disease, an X-linked recessive disease due to the deficiency in the enzyme alpha-galactosidase A which is characterized by angiokeratomas and episodes of pain in the extremities.

The condition is asymptomatic and often an incidental finding. However, patients may be susceptible to glare due to scatter of light by the deposits.

Investigations

(a) A full systemic enquiry will usually uncover the drug in question.
(b) Failure to find a causative drug should lead the clinician to suspect Fabry's disease or other causes of corneal deposits such as chrysiasis (deposition of gold in the stroma) or cystinosis (deposition of cysteine crystals in the stroma, conjunctiva and retinal pigment epithelium).

Management

These deposits are innocuous, need no treatment and are not an indication for the patient to stop drug therapy.

Penetrating keratoplasty

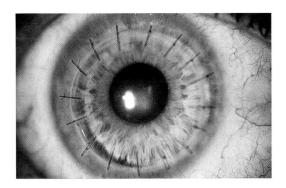

There is a clear centrally sited full-thickness corneal graft or penetrating keratoplasty with 16 interrupted sutures still present. The rest of the eye is normal and there are no abnormalities at the host cornea to suggest the original corneal pathology for which the graft was performed.

The indications for a corneal graft are:

- Optical (such as keratoconus, corneal dystrophy or corneal scarring in an eye with excellent visual potential).
- Tectonic (such as corneal melt or perforation).
- Therapeutic (infective keratitis which is resistant to medical treatment).
- Cosmetic (corneal scarring causing unwanted cosmesis in an eye with no visual potential).

The commonest indications for corneal grafting are secondary endothelial failure such as pseudophakic bullous keratopathy (25%) followed by keratoconus (19%) and primary endothelial failure such as Fuch's endothelial dystrophy.

There are three main types of corneal grafts:

- Epikeratophakia.
- Lamellar keratoplasty.
- Penetrating keratoplasty.

Management

Management of a corneal graft following surgery depends on regular observations to detect and treat any complications which may occur. Complications of penetrating keratoplasty include:

1. Early
   - Haemorrhage or endophthalmitis.
   - Wound leakage causing shallowing of the anterior chamber.
   - Wound dehiscence.

- Corneal oedema due to excessive endothelial loss during surgery.
2.   Late
   - Corneal oedema due to poor donor quality or perioperative loss
   - Wound dehiscence.
   - Postoperative astigmatism.
   - Recurrence of original pathology such as stromal dystrophy in the graft.
   - Graft rejection.
   - Suture abscess.

Tips

Look at the fellow cornea to detect any bilateral corneal conditions such as keratoconus or Fuch's endothelial dystrophy for which the corneal graft was indicated.

Peripheral ulcerative keratitis

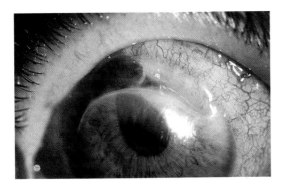

There is an area of thinning at the corneal periphery between 10 and 2 o'clock superiorly with a perforation plugged by iris. The limbal blood vessels are engorged and there are infiltrates at the edge of the ulcer. This is consistent with peripheral ulcerative keratitis (PUK) which can be due to infectious or non-infectious causes.

Differential diagnosis

The non-infectious causes include trauma, neuropathic, keratoconjunctivitis sicca, exposure, Terrien's or Moorens's ulcers and association with systemic vasculitic syndromes such as rheumatoid arthritis, systemic lupus erythematosis, polyarteritis nodosa or Wegener's granulomatosis. Infective causes are usually bacterial in origin.

Investigations

Investigations should be directed to finding the aetiology of the keratitis. An accurate history with an ocular and systemic examination will rule out trauma or infectious causes while providing clues to symptoms and signs of any associated systemic diseases.

Diagnostic tests should include:[1]

(a)   A full blood count.
(b)   An ESR, plasma viscosity or C-reactive protein (an indicator of active vasculitis).
(c)   An autoimmune profile to detect abnormal immune markers such as double-stranded anti-DNA antibody (SLE), rheumatoid factor (rheumatoid arthritis) and antineutrophil cytoplasmic antibody or ANCA (Wegener's).
(d)   A chest X-ray to detect pulmonary lesions in SLE or Wegener's.

Management

Management is directed at the cause. There are two phases of the disease; the active and inactive state.

1. *Inactive state* Here there is peripheral thinning of the cornea but not associated with any symptoms of discomfort and signs of hyperaemia or corneal infiltrate. There is no need for intervention although the patient should be warned of symptoms of active disease which would warrant treatment.

2. *Active disease* This is a serious condition which requires an aggressive combination of medical and surgical intervention especially if PUK is associated with systemic vasculitic diseases or Mooren's ulcer.[1] The therapeutic possibilities are:
   - Systemic and local immunosuppression with steroids.
   - Lid hygiene and ocular lubrication if the condition is associated with a dry eye syndrome.
   - Resection of conjunctiva adjacent to the ulcer to remove the source of collagenase.
   - In this case, where there is corneal perforation, tissue adhesive or a tectonic corneal graft (lamellar or penetrating keratoplasty[2]) may be required to save the eye.

References

1. Sainz de la Maza, M. and Foster, C.S. (1991) The diagnosis and treatment of peripheral ulcerative keratitis. *Semin. Ophthalmol.* **6**, 133–41
2. Foster, C.S. (1980) Immunosuppressive therapy for external ocular inflammatory disease. *Am. J. Ophthal.*, **87**, 140–9

Photorefractive keratectomy (excimer laser)

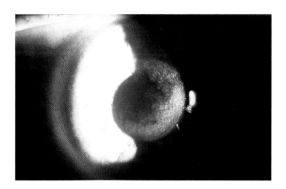

There is 5 mm diameter zone of subepithelial haze in the centre part of the cornea consistent with treatment with excimer laser photorefractive keratectomy (PRK) for myopia. The excimer laser system (which uses argon fluoride) has a wavelength of 193 nm and produces a depth of 0.22 µm with every pulse. Epithelium is removed from the cornea prior to the delivery of laser.

Early complications include pain in the first 24 hours due to the epithelial defect while later the patient may complain of glare due to subepithelial haze, decreased contrast sensitivity, hypermetropia in the first month of treatment and regression towards myopia. Factors such as topical steroids and high preoperative myopia (more than 4 dioptres) may affect the final visual outcome, perhaps by modulating the healing process.

Prognosis

Majority (over 80%) of patients achieve an unaided visual acuity of 6/12 and within 1 dioptre of desired emmetropia.[1,2] Predictability appears best for initial refractive errors less than –4.00 dioptres.

References

1. Ficker, L.A., Bates, A.K., Steele, A.D. McG. (1993) Excimer laser photorefractive keratectomy for myopia: 12 month follow-up. *Eye*, **7**, 617–24
2. Gartry, D.S., Kerr-Muir, M.G. and Marshall, J. (1992) Excimer laser photorefractive keratectomy: 18-month follow-up. *Ophthalmology*, **99**, 1209–19

Interstitial keratitis

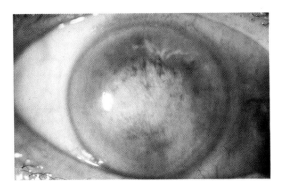

There is central stromal corneal opacity which has radial extensions towards the limbus. Closer examination on higher magnification will reveal 'ghost-vessels'. This is consistent with interstitial keratitis (also described as keratitis linearis migrans) which is most commonly associated with congenital syphilis (luetic disease) along with other causes such as tuberculosis, sarcoidosis and Cogan's disease. The disease begins with an acute corneal inflammation in childhood where the cornea becomes oedematous with subsequent scarring and vascularization. The cornea gradually clears leaving behind a central scar and non-perfused blood vessels ('ghost-vessels') which may refill with blood if the cornea becomes inflamed again. Other signs include thickened Descemet's membrane and linear guttate.

Investigations

(a) There is often a history of ocular inflammation in childhood and there may be other systemic stigmata of luetic disease.

(b) Tuberculosis and sarcoidosis should be excluded with a Mantoux and Kviem test respectively. A chest X-ray may be helpful.

(c) Blood tests such as VDRL and TPHA may reveal markers of luetic disease.

Management

The cause of interstitial keratitis should be established. The treatment depends on the disease activity.

1. In active disease, topical steroids should be given to reduce the inflammatory process. Topical mydriatics will reduce the ciliary spasm secondary to the inflammation. Systemic penicillin is required in active syphilis.[1]

2.   The late manifestation of the disease is an inactive corneal scar. When vision is affected, a penetrating keratoplasty may be required.

Reference

1.   Tamesis, R.R. and Foster, C.S. (1990) Ocular syphilis. *Ophthalmology*, **97**, 1281–7

Corneal foreign body

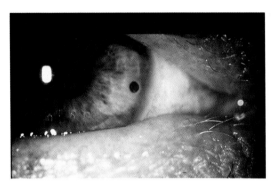

There is a dark round foreign body embedded in the corneal stroma with a ring of brown discoloration around it. This looks like an iron foreign body with a rust ring which is often due to welding sparks or metallic splinters which arise from chiselling or hammering. It causes discomfort or pain, photophobia and lacrimation.

Investigations

(a) An accurate history will differentiate a high-velocity (like hammering) from a low-velocity injury (like welding). This is important as high-velocity projectiles can cause penetrating injuries.

(b) The eye should be examined for other possible foreign bodies, especially beneath the tarsus which requires lid eversion for visualization. A Siedel's test should be performed to exclude aqueous leakage secondary to foreign body penetration. It is important to examine the eye with an indirect ophthalmoscope for a foreign body which may have embedded in the vitreous or retina.

(c) If a metallic intraocular foreign body is suspected, an orbital X-ray will be required.[1] A view with the eyes looking up and another looking down will differentiate between an extraocular (the position of the foreign body does not change) and an intraocular lesion (where it moves with the eye).

Management

1. A superficial foreign body can be easily removed using either a 21-gauge needle or a blade after instilling topical anaesthetic drops.

2. There will be a corneal epithelial defect following this procedure which will require an antibiotic ointment as prophylaxis against infection. The patient should be reviewed once more to ensure complete healing.

References

1. Coleman, D.J., Lucas, B.C., Rondeau, M.J. and Chang, S. (1987) Management of intraocular foreign bodies. *Ophthalmology*, **94**, 1647–53

Herpes simplex disciform scar

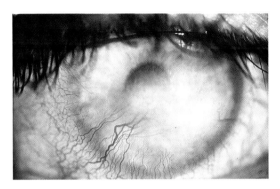

There is a central cornea opacity with a prominent and engorged feeder blood vessel at 7 o'clock. The opacity appears to have an inflammatory infiltrate at 3 o'clock and conjunctival hyperaemia suggestive of an active keratitis around the corneal scar. This is suggestive of a reactivation of herpes simplex keratitis from an old disciform scar. The symptoms experienced are discomfort, photophobia, lacrimation and decreased visual acuity.

Differential diagnosis

Includes an ulcer secondary to an infective cause.

Investigations

(a)   There may be a past history of herpes simplex dendritic ulcer.
(b)   Careful ocular examination is required to detect signs of keratitis (central keratic precipitates and corneal infiltrates) and exclude an active dendritic ulceration (epithelial defect on fluorescein staining) or uveitis (cells and flare in the anterior chamber).
(c)   A conjunctival viral and bacterial swab along with viral serology may help in equivocal cases. In the presence of an ulcer, it is important to exclude a bacterial cause.

Management

It is important to exclude a dendritic ulceration which may be found with the keratitis as this implies active viral replication. This is important as topical steroids should only be used with caution.

1.   *Absence of dendritic ulcer*   In this scenario, weak topical steroids (such as Predsol 0.5% four times daily) are required to reduce the active corneal inflammation which is thought to be an immune reaction to viral antigens. Acyclovir ointment (five times daily) should also be given as prophylaxis.

2.   *Presence of dendritic ulcer*   Acyclovir ointment should be started first to ensure ulcer healing prior to starting weak topical steroids to resolve the keratitis.

Prognosis

It is important to start treatment as early as possible as keratitis leaves behind a scar when the active inflammation has resolved. Future episodes of reactivation may occur and may require regular topical weak steroids (once or alternate daily) as prophylaxis. If the scar is extensive, the patient will require a penetrating keratoplasty to improve vision.[1]

Reference

1.   Ficker, L.A., Kirkness, C.M., Rice, N.S.C. and Steele, A.D.McG. (1989) The changing management and improved prognosis for corneal grafting in herpes simplex keratitis. *Ophthalmology*, **96**, 1587–96

Conjunctiva/sclera

Scleromalacia perforans

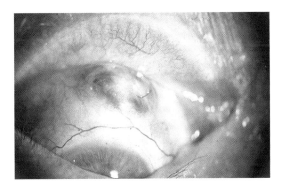

There is an area of scleral thinning superiorly behind the limbus with underlying uvea visible in an otherwise quiet eye. This is consistent with scleromalacia perforans (also called anterior necrotizing scleritis without inflammation). The condition is found most commonly in women within the ages of 60–70 years. It is associated with systemic diseases in around 50% of cases such as connective tissue disorders (rheumatoid arthritis, systemic lupus erythematosis, polyarteritis nodosa, sarcoidosis, Wegener's granulomatosis) and infections like herpes zoster, tuberculosis and syphilis.

There are two types of scleritis and each type has varying presentations:[1]

1. **Anterior scleritis** which can be either necrotizing or non-necrotizing.
   - Non-necrotizing scleritis presents as a hyperaemic eye with ocular discomfort and photophobia. On examination, there are two patterns of inflammation, the nodular and the diffuse pattern which can be mistaken as episcleritis.
   - Necrotizing scleritis can occur either with an inflammatory response (an intensely hyperaemic eye with extreme pain, photophobia and nausea) or without one when the patient is often asymptomatic and the eye quiet.
2. **Posterior scleritis** accounts for 10–20% of scleritis cases. It gives rise to retrobulbar pain and causes visual disturbance if it is complicated by uveal effusion syndrome, serous retinal detachment or choroidal effusion secondary to the inflammation.

Investigations

(a) Systemic examination to exclude underlying systemic diseases. This includes a FBC, ESR, VDRL, chest X-ray and an immunological profile for rheumatoid factor and other markers of autoimmune disease such as antineutrophil cytoplasmic autoantibodies (ANCA) in Wegener's granulomatosis.

(b)   Fundal examination to exclude retinal complications.
(c)   US or MRI may help delineate the extent of scleritis from the thickness of the sclera.
(d)   FFA may be helpful in detecting areas of scleral hypoperfusion in narcotizing scleritis.

Management[2]

As scleritis is nearly always an ocular manifestation of a systemic disorder, the treatment is always systemic although topical lubricants and steroids may play a role in keeping the eye comfortable.

1.   Non-necrotizing scleritis can be treated with non-steroidal anti-inflammatory drugs (NSAID) alone. A good NSAID is oxyphenbutazone 600 mg daily initially and then reducing to 400 mg daily when the inflammation has improved. Indomethacin 100 mg and reducing to 75 mg daily on clinical improvement is an alternative.
2.   Necrotizing scleritis is a serious disease and requires prompt high-dose immunosuppression to control the inflammatory process. Immunosuppression can be with oral steroids (60–80 mg prednisolone initially and then reduce gradually with clinical improvement) or steroid-sparing drugs such as azathioprine or cyclophosphamide.[3]

Note that it is important to ensure that these patients do not have evidence of gastric erosions or ulcers before commencing treatment with steroids or NSAIDs. An H_2-antagonist such as ranitidine or cimetidine may be required to protect the gastric mucosa.

Prognosis

It is important to exclude a systemic disease associated with scleritis, especially Wegener's granulomatosis, as it carries an 82% mortality rate within one year due to renal complications if the disease is not treated with immunosuppression.

References

1.   Tuft, S. and Watson, P.G. (1991) Progression of scleral disease. *Ophthalmology*, **98**, 467–71
2.   Watson, P.G. (1980) The diagnosis and management of scleritis. *Ophthalmology*, **87**, 716–20.
3.   Foster, C.S. (1980) Immunosuppression therapy for external ocular inflammatory disease. *Ophthalmology*, **87**, 140–50

Allergic conjunctivitis

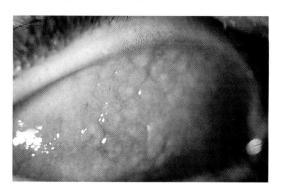

There is a 'velvet-like' pinkish chemotic conjunctiva with 'ropey' mucus and fine papillary reaction (defn: micropapillae <0.3 mm, macropapillae 0.3–1 mm, giant papillae >1 mm) on upper and lower tarsal conjunctiva. There is no purulent discharge nor follicles suggestive of bacterial and viral cause. The findings are consistent with an allergic conjunctivitis.

Differential diagnosis

Includes blepharoconjunctivitis, superior limbic keratoconjunctivitis, bacterial, viral and cicatricial conjunctivitis.

Investigations

(a) A history of exposure to allergen (dust-mites, fur and ragweed pollen), topical medication and contact-lens wear points towards an allergic cause especially when the patient has a family history of atopy such as asthma and eczema.
(b) Conjunctival scrapings for Gram and Giemsa (characterizes inflammatory cellular response with lymphocytic predominance in viral and trachoma, eosinophils in allergy, polymorphonuclear cells in bacterial infection) stains, and a swab for cultures.
(c) There may be an increase in serum and tear levels of IgE and eosinophils.

Management

This depends on the type of allergic conjunctivitis.[1]

1. *Seasonal allergic (hay-fever) rhinoconjunctivitis* Avoidance of airborne allergens (e.g. regular changing of bed-linen) which results in an IgE-mediated type 1 hypersensitivity reaction with release of histamine, prostaglandins from mast cells.[2] Allergens may be identified by skin patch testing. Systemic and topical antihistamines such

as sodium cromoglycate, lodoxamide and nedocromil may prevent mast cell degranulation by stabilizing cell membranes.

2. *Atopic keratoconjunctivitis*   Occurs in males between ages 30 and 50 years with family history of atopy (asthma, eczema, hay fever). In addition, there may be conjunctival scarring, punctate corneal keratitis, blepharitis and lid dermatitis. Manage as in (1). In addition, weak topical steroids may be needed during acute attacks to avoid corneal and conjunctival complications.

3. *Vernal keratoconjunctivitis*   Occurs in boys and girls between the ages of 6 and 20 years, with an initial predominance in boys. Majority have a family history of atopy although 10% are non-atopic. Limbal vernal with Horner–Trantas' dots is more common in black patients. Beware corneal changes such as punctate epithelial keratitis of Togby, mucus plaque ulcer, sub-epithelial scarring and pseudo gerontoxon.[2] Manage as in (2).

4. *Giant papillary (>1 mm papillae) conjunctivitis*   Discontinue contact lens (usually soft type).

5. *Contact allergic conjunctivitis*   Discontinue known allergen, which usually precedes reaction by 4–10 hours.

Tips

Dermatological abnormalities on the face associated with allergy such as acne rosacea, scratch marks, periorbital oedema and Dennies's line (fold of skin on the lower eyelid) may be present.

References

1. Buckley, R.J. (1993) Allergic conjunctivitis. *Survey of Ophthalmology*, **38** (Suppl.), 105–14
2. Buckley, R.J. (1988) Vernal conjunctivitis. *International Ophthalmic Clinics*, **28**, 303–8

Chemical burn

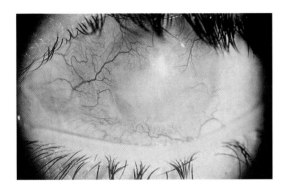

There is extensive opacification and vascularization of the cornea with both deep and superficial vessels invading from all around the limbus. This is consistent with severe corneal scarring associated with a chemical (especially alkali such as ammonia, lime and wet cement) burn. Other late complications include persistent corneal epithelial defect, dry eye, symblepharon formation, cicatricial entropion, uveitis and even corneal melt leading to perforation in a severe burn. The Roper–Hall classification helps to assess the prognosis of the eye following a chemical burn.

Grade	Clinical findings	Prognosis
1	Epithelial damage without limbal ischaemia	Good
2	Hazy cornea but iris still visible. Limbal ischaemia <1/3	Good
3	Total loss of corneal epithelium. Stromal oedema obscures iris details. Limbal ischaemia between 1/3-1/2	Guarded
4	Opaque cornea. Limbal ischaemia >1/2	Poor

Investigations

(a) The diagnosis is a clinical one and a detailed history will uncover the aetiological factor for the scarring.

(b) The pH of the offending chemical can be tested with a pH paper placed on the inferior fornix.

Management

Prompt diagnosis and intervention is required.[1]

1. *Immediate* The eye should have copious irrigation for at least 5–10 minutes with the nearest available source of running water such as a tap or shower. This water should preferably be clean to prevent

the risk of secondary infection. The patient should then be transferred immediately to an eye hospital.

2. *Early*   At the hospital, topical anaesthetic should be applied and an eyelid speculum inserted for further irrigation with sterile solutions such as Hartmann's solution. The pH is checked at intervals to ensure the eye achieves a neutral pH before stopping irrigation for a complete ocular examination to assess the extent of damage. The treatment for minor (grade 1) burns consists of prophylactic topical antibiotics and cycloplegics to prevent ciliary spasm during the healing period. The epithelial defect should heal within a few days. More severe burns require admission for more intensive treatment which consists of a combination of the following:

   - Topical antibiotics as prophylaxis.
   - Topical steroids (dexamethasone 4 times daily) to reduce the inflammatory process on the conjunctiva or anterior chamber which accompanies grade 2/3 burns.
   - Topical 10% and systemic (1-2 g daily) ascorbic acid may be useful as it helps in collagen repair and is a natural scavenger of free radicals.
   - Drugs to reduce any rise in IOP which may occur.

3. *Late*   treatment depends on the complications (see above) which may arise. Dry eye should be treated like any case of keratoconjunctivitis sicca while cicatricial entropion and corneal melt have already been discussed elsewhere in this book. Persistent corneal epithelial defect occurs due to the loss of limbal 'stem cells' following limbal ischaemia. A limbal autologous conjunctival transplantation may repopulate these cells when harvested from the fellow eye. The opaque cornea is due to a combination of stromal vascularization and oedema. A corneal penetrating keratoplasty may be an option but faces a definite high risk of corneal rejection due to the presence of deep vessels in the stroma.

Prognosis

Visual rehabilitation is often poor due to problems mentioned above.

Reference

1. Ragge, N.K. and Easty, D.L. (1990). *Immediate Eye Care*. Wolfe Publishing, London, pp. 245–52

Pterygium

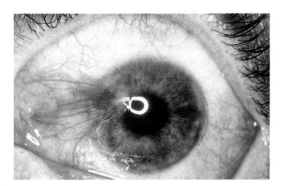

This is a fleshy fibrovascular lesion originating from the nasal conjunctiva encroaching the cornea at the 3 o'clock position but sparing the visual axis by 3 mm. Anatomically there are three parts to the lesion; the cap (halo-like avascular zone at the front), the head and the body. This is consistent with a pterygium associated with ageing, hot and dry climates. Other signs include either dellen formation or iron deposition (Stocker's line) at the leading edge of the lesion, with-the-rule astigmatism and restriction of horizontal ocular movements.

Differential diagnosis

Includes a pseudopterygium (associated with chemical burns, cicatricial diseases, marginal ulcers) and conjunctival tumour.

Management

Management can be either observation if it is asymptomatic, or surgery if the lesion is symptomatic, cosmetically unacceptable and encroaching the visual axis. The surgical options are:

1. Excision of the lesion leaving the conjunctival defect bare (the 'bare sclera technique').
2. Excision and superficial keratectomy (when the pterygium covers the cornea) followed by a lamellar corneal graft to cover the corneal defect.

To reduce the risk of recurrence, adjunctive therapy may be applied to the conjunctival defect after surgery. Options include:

- Beta-radiation.
- Instillation of anti-mitotic agents such as mitomycin-C.
- Closure of the defect with either a free or rotational conjunctival autograft.

Prognosis

The recurrence rates vary from 14% using conjunctival autografting to 80% with a bare scleral technique.[1]

Tip

A true pterygium is adherent to the underlying structure throughout while a pseudopterygium is fixed, usually at the apex. This can be demonstrated by looping under the lesion with a squint hook.

Reference

1. Riordan-Eva, P., Kielhorn, I., Ficker, L.A. *et al.* (1993) Conjunctival autografting in the surgical management of pterygium. *Eye*, **7**, 634–8

Cicatricial entropion

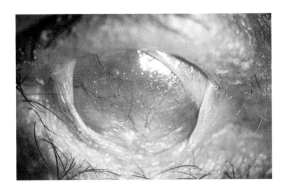

There is a symblepharon with loss of the inferior fornix in the lower lid which appears to be turning in. This is consistent with a cicatricial entropion due to cicatricial pemphigoid which is a bilateral auto-immune disease characterized by recurrent blisters of mucous membranes affecting middle-aged women.

Other features which can be found include ankyloblepharon (adhesions between the eyelids), trichiasis (in-turning eyelashes), distichiasis (abnormally sited lashes), poor tear film due to keratoconjunctivitis sicca and xerophthalmia, scarring of the punctum and corneal changes secondary to exposure and poor tear film.

Differential diagnosis

Includes chemical (especially alkali) burns, Stevens–Johnson syndrome and iatrogenic causes (following radiotherapy, topical drugs such as Ganda, pilocarpine, adrenaline and systemic practolol).

Investigations

(a) A thorough history of medication should be taken.
(b) A systemic examination to assess the involvement of other mucous membrane sites in pemphigoid such as the oral and nasal cavities, oesophagus and anus, and vagina. These lesions may heal leaving smooth atrophic scars.

There are four stages to ocular pemphigoid:[1]

- Conjunctival inflammation.
- Conjunctival shrinkage (especially the inferior fornix).
- Advanced shrinkage (symblepharon, corneal vascularization).
- End-stage (ankyloblepharon, corneal keratinization, severe sicca syndrome).

Management

1. *Acute*   During the inflammatory phase of the disease, systemic and topical immunosuppresion should be given in high doses.
2. *Late/chronic*   During this stage, the treatment is aimed at keeping the eye comfortable and the prevention of corneal problems such as ulceration, erosions and infections.
    *   Conservative: such measures include artificial tears and ointment, moist chambers, regular lid hygiene, epilation for trichiasis and early intervention in the event of secondary infections.
    *   Surgery: when lid changes such as cicatricial entropion threaten to affect the cornea, surgery should be undertaken to evert the lid. The options are either anterior lamellar repositioning, posterior lamellar graft or mucous membrane graft.

Prognosis

Although aggressive intervention at the early stage may limit the extent of damage to the ocular structures, at the late stage the outlook is poor and requires considerable effort to keep the eye comfortable and free of complications.

Reference

1. Foster, C.S., Wilson, L.A. and Ekins, M.B. (1982) Immunosuppressive therapy for progressive ocular cicatricial pemphigoid. *Ophthalmology*, **89**, 340–53

Intraepithelial conjunctival tumour

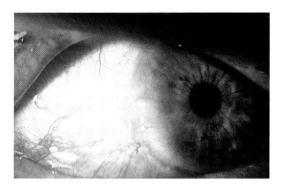

There is a conjunctival flat lesion at the nasal aspect of the globe which is encroaching the cornea. It has blood vessels on it and appears attached to the underlying sclera and cornea.

Differential diagnosis

Includes intraepithelial conjunctival tumour (also known as carcinoma-in-situ, Bowen's disease or intraepithelial epithelioma), squamous cell carcinoma of conjunctiva, conjunctival amelanotic naevus, papilloma, lymphangioma, lipoma or myxoma.

Investigations

(a) A careful examination under high magnification may help. Staining with a dye such as fluorescein or Rose Bengal can outline the outer limit of the tumour.

(b) A tissue biopsy may be required. This is particularly important when differentiating between intraepithelial tumour (whereby the tumour is confined to the epithelial layer) and squamous cell carcinoma (where the dysplastic process breaks through the basement membrane).

This case was in fact an intraepithelial conjunctival tumour, which is associated with exposure to chemical, radiation or harsh weather conditions. The role of viruses such as herpes simplex and papilloma virus is uncertain.

Management

1. The treatment is surgical. The edge of the tumour should be outlined in theatre with dye prior to surgery. The options are either freezing

or excision although it appears that a combination of freezing and excision has a lower rate of recurrence.[1] Histological confirmation should be obtained. If the tumour involves the cornea or sclera, a superficial keratectomy or sclerectomy should be performed to remove as much tumour as possible.

2. The patient should be seen regularly to detect evidence of recurrence.

Prognosis

The rate of recurrence varies from 20 to 40%, although combination treatment of excision and freezing is associated with a recurrence rate of only 8%. Complications of treatment include superficial scarring and pannus formation.

Reference

1. Fraunfelder, F.T. and Wingfield, D. (1983) Management of intraepithelial conjunctival tumours and squamous cell carcinomas. *American Journal of Ophthalmology*, **95**, 359–63

Conjunctival naevus

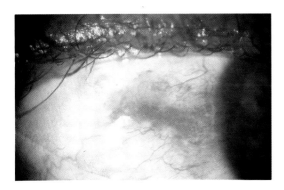

There is a lesion at the limbus which is raised and fleshy with variable pigmentation and cyst formation. This is consistent with a conjunctival junctional naevus. Histologically the lesion consists of dendritic shaped melanocytes but may have atypical cytology as naevi have malignant potential and may give rise to a melanoma.[1]

Differential diagnosis

Includes primary acquired melanosis (PAM), conjunctival melanoma and pigmented squamous cell carcinoma which may have similar appearances.

Investigations[2]

(a) An accurate history will reveal the time onset of the lesion and any recent change in its size. The lesion should also be photographed as documentation of its size and shape.
(b) If there is doubt and PAM is suspected, the lesion should be biopsied. Cytological atypia is more likely to give rise to a melanoma.

Management

1. All suspicious lesions should be biopsied.
2. A lesion with cytological atypia or which shows a rapid rate of growth should be surgically excised completely with further adjuvant therapy of either:
    • Cryotherapy.
    • Beta-radiation or external beam radiotherapy.

Prognosis

There is risk of a naevus becoming a melanoma. Melanomas with a poor prognosis include those with a thickness of more than 1 mm (with a mortality of around 33–50%), caruncular melanomas, lymphatic invasion and mitotic activity.

References

1. Yanoff, M. and Fine, B.S. *Ocular Pathology*, 2nd edn, Gower Medical Publishing, New York
2. Folberg, R., McLean, I.W. and Zimmerman, L.E. (1984) Conjunctival melanosis and melanoma. *Ophthalmology*, **91**, 673–8

Conjunctival pigment deposits

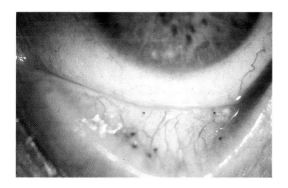

There are conjunctival pigment deposits on the inferior tarsal conjunctiva. This is an example of non-melanocytic pigmentation which can be due to a variety of causes. Deposits can be due to endogenous pigmentation in ochronosis, Wilson's and Addison's disease or secondary to exogenous pigmentation such as foreign body (mascara or dust particles), argyrosis, chrysiasis or long-term use of adrenalin.

Investigations

(a) Using a cotton-bud, foreign bodies can be easily removed.
(b) Exclude melanocytic causes such as conjunctival epithelial melanosis, naevus or melanoma by careful examination. If necessary, a biopsy may be required.

Management

1. Non-melanocytic pigmentation is benign and requires no treatment.
2. It is essential that melanocytic causes such as conjunctival epithelial melanosis, naevus or melanoma are excluded.

Ocular melanocytosis

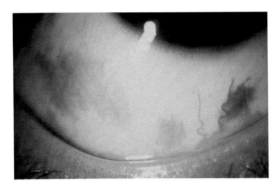

There is increased pigmentation of the sclera and episclera in the eye of this patient. The overlying conjunctiva is mobile and not attached to these lesions. This is consistent with ocular melanocytosis (or melanosis oculi) which is unilateral and more commonly found in blacks and Orientals with an incidence of 0.1–0.5%. These lesions are often present at birth but may appear later in life with a propensity to increase in size and colour at around puberty. There may be increased pigmentation of the uveal tract resulting in heterochromia. It may be associated with increased pigmentation of the skin in the distribution of the ophthalmic or maxillary division of the cranial nerve; this is called oculodermal melanocytosis or naevus of Ota. Histologically, the lesions are composed of hyperpigmented melanocytes. There is an increased risk in developing uveal melanomas.

Investigations

(a) Both eyes should be examined. In view of the increased risk of developing uveal tumours, the fundus should be assessed.

(b) Other causes of pigmentation of the external eye and conjunctiva (such as conjunctival melanosis) should be excluded. If in doubt, a tissue biopsy should be taken.

Management

The patient should be made aware of the increased risk of developing uveal tumours and therefore should be examined at regular intervals.[1]

Reference

1. Velaquez, N. and Jones, I.S. (1983) Ocular and oculodermal melanocytosis associated with uveal melanoma. *Ophthalmology*, **90**, 1472–6

Iris, lens and anterior chamber

Pigment dispersion syndrome

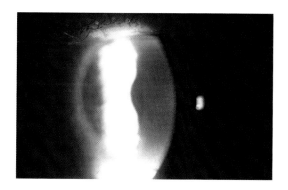

There is pigment deposition vertically on the corneal endothelium (Krukenberg spindle) with spoke-like mid-iris pigment epithelium defects on transillumination and pigment deposition (Scheie stripe) on the lens (and zonules if the pupil is well-dilated). The iris bows posteriorly at the periphery thus the postulate that pigment is dispersed when the iris rubs against the zonules. This is consistent with pigment dispersion syndrome and is associated with raised intraocular pressure (pigmentary glaucoma) in 50% of cases.[1] It characteristically affects young myopic (around -3 dioptres) Caucasian males.

Differential diagnosis

Includes pseudoexfoliation syndrome (which has transillumination defects in the pupillary ruff), pseudophakics with IOL in contact with the iris, pigment release from a primary uveal melanoma or oculodermal melanocytosis and bloodstaining of cornea.

Investigations

(a) A gonioscopy will confirm pigment on zonule and trabecular meshwork (Sampaolesi's line), and exclude presence of pseudoexfoliation material.

(b) The anterior chamber may be deeper than normal on biometric measurements.

Management[2]

1. Regular observation is sufficient as only 50% will develop pigmentary glaucoma.

2. Should intraocular pressure rise, long-term control may be difficult as the disease begins at an early age. Initially, medical treatment should be given as for any open angle glaucoma. Miotics are thought

to work by decreasing irido-zonular apposition. Argon laser trabeculoplasty works well while drainage surgery tends to fare badly.

Prognosis

Difficult to control IOP, although this condition is thought to improve with age.

Tips

Check fellow eye for bilaterality of condition. Look for evidence of previous drainage or laser surgery.

References

1. Farrar, S.M., Shields, M.B., Miller, K.N. and Stoup, C.M. (1989) Risk factors for the development and severity of glaucoma in the pigment dispersion syndrome. *American Journal of Ophthalmology*, **108,** 223–9
2. Farrar, S.M. and Shields, M.B. (1993) Current concepts in pigmentary glaucoma. *Survey of Ophthalmology*, **37**, 233–52

Fuch's heterochromic uveitis

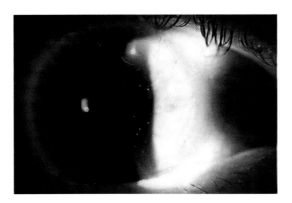

There is heterochromia present with presence of stellate non-pigmented keratic precipitates scattered throughout the corneal endothelium. Other signs include slight anterior chamber activity, abnormal iris vessels which extend to the angle and are prone to bleeding (Amsler's sign) in the eye with the hypochromic (washed-out appearance) atrophic iris. This is consistent with Fuch's heterochromic uveitis, a unilateral condition which is associated with the development of cataract and secondary open angle glaucoma (in 25%) in the affected eye. It accounts for 1.5–3% of the uveitis population.

Differential diagnosis

The differential diagnosis of heterochromia includes:

- Hypochromia – congenital simple; congenital Horner's; association with Duane's; Posner–Schlossman syndrome; chronic uveitis; pigment dispersion syndrome; Waardenburg's syndrome.
- Hyperchromia – melanosis; iris naevus syndrome; xanthochromia; siderosis.

Investigations

(a) This should be directed at excluding other causes of heterochromia, especially the presence of intraocular metallic (iron) foreign body.
(b) Anterior segment fluorescein angiogram is not required but will reveal abnormal iris vessel fronds and sectoral atrophy.

Management

Management of the condition is directed at three areas:[1]

(1) *Uveitis* – Needs no treatment unless uveitis is severe as steroids may cause steroid-induced glaucoma and cataracts.

(2)   *Glaucoma* – Difficult to manage but treat as open-angle glaucoma. Bleb failure is common after surgical drainage and may require adjunct therapy.[2]

(3)   *Cataract* – Although controversial in the 1960s, cataract extraction is considered a safe surgical option. The risk of postoperative uveitis is higher in eyes with severe iris atrophy but may be reduced with the use of heparin surface-modified IOL and more intensive topical steroids postoperatively.

Prognosis

Good, although glaucoma may be difficult to manage.

Tip

Heterochromia is best appreciated with daylight.

References

1.   Jones, N.P. (1991) Fuch's heterochromic uveitis. A reappraisal of the clinical spectrum. *Eye*, **5**, 649–61
2.   Heuer, D.K., Parrish, R.K., Gressel, M.G. *et al.* (1986) 5-Fluorouracil and glaucoma filtering surgery. Intermediate follow-up of a pilot study. *Ophthalmology*, **93**, 1537–46

Ocular siderosis

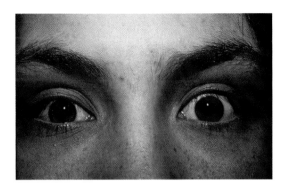

There is heterochromia with the darker eye showing pupillary mydriasis and iron deposition on the endothelium. This is consistent with ocular siderosis due to retention of iron-containing intraocular foreign body (IOFB) following a penetrating injury.[1] Other signs include iron deposition beneath the lens capsule, lens opacification, pigmentary glaucoma, retinal pigmentary change and phthsis bulbi at the later stages.

Differential diagnosis

The differential diagnosis of heterochromia includes:
- Hypochromia – congenital simple; congenital Horner's; association with Duane's; Posner–Schlossman syndrome; chromic uveitis; pigment dispersion syndrome; Waardenburg's syndrome.
- Hyperchromia – melanosis; iris naevus syndrome; xanthochromia.

Investigations

(a) A skull X-ray and CT scan may detect the presence of a metallic IOFB.

(b) Electroretinogram (ERG) shows deterioration with a gradual reduction in the B-wave with time as a consequence of the toxic effect of iron retention.

(c) Light microscopy of the tissue shows widespread iron deposition (using Perl's stain) in non-pigmented retinal epithelium and conjunctiva.

Management[2]

All IOFBs should be removed at the early stages. However, the choice of treatment is controversial. If a foreign body is found later when visual acuity remains stable, surgical intervention may be complicated by proliferative vitreoretinopathy postoperatively. The choices are:

1.   Serial electrophysiology to follow retained IOFB and removal considered when deterioration is detected.
2.   Surgical intervention which may either be:
   - Sclerostomy and removal with a magnet.
   - Pars plana vitrectomy and removal with IOFB forceps.

Tips

1.   Retained IOFB is usually found in the inferior aspect of the eye.
2.   Look for entry sites which may prove positive on Siedel's test.
3.   The eye may be soft.

References

1.   Hope-Ross, M., Mahon, G.J. and Johnson, P.B. (1993) Ocular siderosis. *Eye*, **7**, 419–25
2.   Sneed, R.S. and Weingeist, T.A. (1990) Management of siderosis bulbi due to a retained iron containing intraocular foreign body. *Ophthalmology*, **97**, 375–9

Primary open angle glaucoma

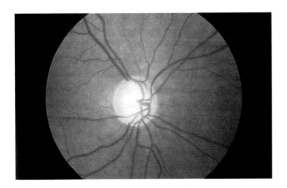

There is a pale, thinned neuroretinal rim around a cupped disc with a cup disc ratio of 0.7 and superior notching resulting in displacement of the vessels nasally and 'bayoneting' of the vessel as it enters the disc.

Differential diagnosis

Differential diagnosis of a cupped disc includes open (and narrow) angle glaucoma, normal tension glaucoma, anterior ischaemic optic neuropathy, compressive lesion on the optic nerve or benign intracranial hypertension.

Investigations

(a) Full ocular examination of the cornea (megalocornea and Haab's striae suggest congenital glaucoma while corneal oedema is present with very high IOP), angle (to discriminate between open and narrow angles by measuring the angle using Shaffer, Spaeth or Van Herick's method of grading and to detect pigmentation of the trabeculum in pigmentary glaucoma), iris (naevus/atrophy in iridocorneal syndrome, evidence of glaucoma surgery such as laser iridotomies/iridectomy, rubeotic vessels, iris atrophy and spiral suggests previous acute narrow angle glaucomatous attack) and lens (which may be involved in phacogenic glaucoma).

(b) Tonometry to measure systolic IOP or 24 hour phasing to identify peaks over 21 mm/Hg.

(c) Perimetry to detect field defects such as extension of the blind spot, scotomas within 10–20° fixation (Bjerrum area), arcuate field defect (Seidel scotoma), arcuate defect which coalesces with the blind spot (Bjerrum scotoma), nasal step (Roenne) and temporal wedge.

Management

Management of primary open angle glaucoma in essence involves medical, laser and surgical treatment to lower IOP and preserve visual field. Controversy arises over the order of preference.[1]

1.   Medical treatment
     - Parasympathomimetics – pilocarpine or phospholine iodide.
     - Adrenergic agonists – epinephrine and dipivalyl epinephrine (propine), a prodrug of epinephrine.
     - Beta-adrenergic blocking drugs.
     - Carbonic anhydrase inhibitors (CAI) such as acetazolamide and methazolamide may be required to reduce IOP rapidly or while waiting for surgery when topical therapy has failed.
2.   Laser treatment
     - Argon laser trabeculoplasty.
     - Laser sclerostomy.
3.   Surgical treatment of choice is a trabeculectomy. It can be in conjunction with antimitotic drugs (such as mitomycin C or 5-fluorouracil) if there is a high risk of failure due to scarring, especially in the young age group and Negro races. Molteno tube implant may be required if all else fails.
4.   Ciliary body ablation (trans-scleral YAG laser and cyclocryotherapy). The indications are end-stage failed filter, neovascularization and silicone oil induced glaucoma.

Tips

All glaucoma patients should be followed-up regularly to detect any progression of disease. Also look for disc haemorrhages, reduced neuroretinal layer seen with red-free light, pores within the lamina cribosa and examine the disc in the fellow eye.

Reference

1.   Dutton, J. and Slamovits, T. (1993) Initial treatment of glaucoma: surgery or medications. Viewpoints. *Survey of Ophthalmology*, **37**, 293–305

Pseudoexfoliation syndrome

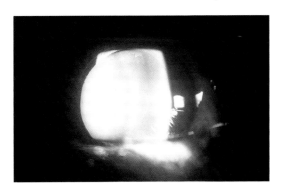

There is greyish-white flaky material circumferentially at the periphery and centre of the anterior lens capsule with a 'tide-mark' pattern. This is consistent with deposition of proteoglycan (amyloid-like) material in pseudoexfoliation syndrome (PXE). It affects the elderly population, especially in the Greek and Scandinavian population, and is bilateral in half the cases. Around 60% of patients develop raised intraocular pressure leading to glaucoma. Other signs include deposition of the material on the pupillary margins, angle and zonules, iris atrophy at the mid-periphery which transilluminates, hyperpigmentation of the trabecular meshwork (Sampaolesi's line) and cupped discs.[1]

Investigations

(a) The intraocular pressure (IOP) should be measured, angle viewed with a gonioscope and the disc examined in both eyes. The PXE material is better seen with the pupil dilated.
(b) The visual fields should be examined for any scotomas.

Management

The management is identical to that in open angle glaucoma (OAG) in the presence of raised intraocular pressure and PXE. The options are:

1. Medications such as topical beta-blockers and miotics.
2. Laser trabeculoplasty appears to be effective.[2]
3. Surgery (trabeculectomy).

Prognosis

Like other secondary OAGs, the IOP is usually more difficult to control than in primary OAG. As such, these patients should be seen on a regular basis (6- to 9-monthly) to ensure that any deterioration in the condition will be detected early.

References

1.   Konstas, A.G.P., Jay, J.L., Marshall, G.E. and Lee, W.R. (1993) Prevalence, diagnostic features and response to trabeculectomy in exfoliation glaucoma. *Ophthalmology*, **100**, 619–27
2.   Coakes, R. (1992) Laser trabeculoplasty. *British Journal of Ophthalmology*, **76**, 624–6

Rubeosis irides

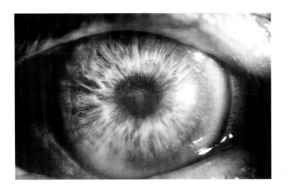

There is a collection of small blood vessels around the sphincter of the iris radiating to the periphery. The cornea is clear and devoid of oedema, and the angle deep without peripheral anterior synechiae.

Differential diagnosis

Includes normal dilated tuft of iris vasculature or rubeosis irides secondary to ischaemia such as central retinal vein occlusion, proliferative diabetic retinopathy, necrotic intraocular tumours or chronic retinal detachment.[1]

Investigations

Investigation should involve a full ocular examination to find the cause. It should include:

(a) Gonioscopy which will detect new vessels in the angle.
(b) Complete fundal examination.

Management

Management should be directed at the cause, like CRVO and DM, whereby panretinal argon photocoagulation may reverse rubeosis at the early stages.[2] At the late stage, when there is no useful vision remaining, the aim is to keep the eye comfortable and free of corneal oedema by reducing IOP via:

1. Medical means
    • Adrenergic agonists such as epinephrine and dipivalyl pinephrine (propine).
    • Beta-adrenergic blocking drugs.
    • Carbonic anhydrase inhibitors (CAI) such as acetazolamide and methazolamide.

2.   Ciliary body ablation (trans-scleral YAG laser and cyclocryother-
      apy).
3.   Surgical means
      • Trabeculectomy with adjuvant anti-fibrotic agents.
      • Molteno tube implant.

The eye, meanwhile, can be kept comfortable by maintaining a dilated
pupil with topical atropine. An end-stage painful rubeotic eye may leave
the surgeon no option but to enucleate.

Reference

1.   Henkind, P. (1978) Ocular neovascularisation. The Krill Memorial Lecture.
      American Journal of Ophthalmology, **85**, 287–301
2.   The Diabetic Retinopathy Study Research Group. (1978) Photocoagulation
      treatment of proliferative diabetic retinopathy: the second report of diabetic
      retinopathy study findings. *Ophthalmology*, **85**, 82–106

Aniridia

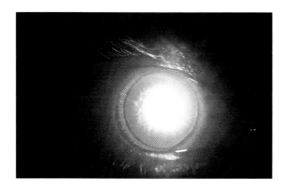

There is almost complete absence of iris in both eyes. This is consistent with aniridia with an incidence of 1 in 90 000. Other features seen are foveal, optic nerve or macula hypoplasia, pendular nystagmus, secondary glaucoma, corneal pannus, epidermal dermoids, cataract and lens subluxation.[1] Systemic associations include Wilm's tumour, genitourinary system abnormalities and mental retardation. There are three genetic types of aniridia:

- Sporadic cases of which two-thirds represent a fresh dominant mutation (AN1).
- Autosomal dominant (AN2).
- Autosomal recessive (AN3).

Investigations

(a) Full family history and general examination.
(b) Full ocular examination to exclude treatable complications such as glaucoma and cataract.

Management

The condition should be managed in conjunction with a paediatrician.
1. Genetic counselling.
2. Regular systemic examination and renal ultrasound until the age of 8 years to exclude the development of a Wilm's tumour.
3. Glaucoma should be treated, although the control of IOP may be difficult.
4. Tinted glasses or iris occluders may be useful to reduce photophobia.

Reference

1. Johns, K.J. and O'Day, D.M. (1991) Posterior chamber intraocular lenses after extracapsular cataract extraction in patients with aniridia. *Ophthalmology*, **98**, 1698–702

Albinism

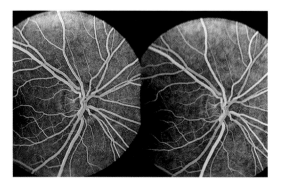

Albinism is due to the failure of melanin production. There are two types of albinism.[1]

- Oculo-cutaneous albinism, which has an autosomal recessive inheritance and is characterized by hypomelanosis of the hair, skin and eye.
- Ocular albinism, where the hypomelanosis is confined to the eyes only. This can either be of autosomal or more commonly X-linked recessive (also known as Nettleship–Falls) inheritance. The female carriers may show iris translucency and characteristic 'mud-splattered' areas of depigmentation in the fundus.[2] The affected males have poor vision, refractive errors, iris translucency, fundal hypopigmentation, foveal hypoplasia, strabismus and nystagmus. Although they have no clinical skin involvement, skin biopsy may show the presence of giant melanin granules or macromelanosomes.

Management

1. Genetic counselling. Examination of the patient's mother (fundus and iris) is important in the detection of her carrier status.
2. There is no effective treatment.

Prognosis

The X-linked recessively inherited ocular albinism has the best final visual acuity (6/18–6/60) compared to the oculocutaneous type where visual acuity is rarely better than 6/60.

Reference

1. Kinnear, P.E., Jay, B. and Witcop, C.J. Jr (1985) Albinism. *Survey of Ophthalmology*, **30**, 75–101.
2. Charles, S.J., Moore, A.J., Grant, J.W. and Yates, J.W.R. (1992) Genetic counselling in X-linked ocular albinism: clinical features in the carrier state. *Eye*, **6**, 75–9

Iris melanoma

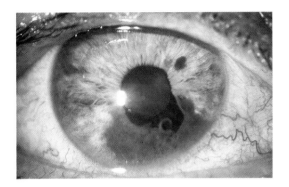

There is a pigmented lesion at the inferior aspect of the iris with prominent intrinsic blood vessels, ectropion irides and secondary sectoral cataract. It is suggestive of an iris melanoma and is associated with light coloured iris in Caucasians in the fourth decade. Iris melanoma accounts for 3–10% of all malignant melanomas of the uvea.

Differential diagnosis

Includes iris naevus (which occur *de novo* or in conjunction with Cogan–Reese and ICE syndromes), iris cyst (which may have a history of trauma or topical miotics or foreign body[1]), leiomyoma, neurofibroma or a metastatic lesion (10% of ocular metastasis involve the iris).

Investigations

(a) A 3-mirror gonioscopic evaluation to exclude involvement of the angle and ciliary body.
(b) Anterior fluorescein angiography shows diffuse confluent fluorescence.
(c) Radioactive phosphorous uptake and ultrasonography may be helpful.

Management

Management may involve doing nothing but regular observation of the lesion if it is static and the patient declines surgical intervention, especially when the vision is unaffected. Only 5% of such lesions show growth within 5 years of diagnosis. However, should surgery be required, the options depends on the size and extent of the tumour.[2]

1. Iridectomy if the involvement is less than 5 clock hours.
2. Iridocyclectomy if the angle is involved.

3.   Enucleation if the lesion is an iris ring melanoma involving more than 50% circumference or if it causes pain or raised intraocular pressure.

Prognosis

Excellent, with a 5-year mortality of less than 5%.

Tips

Look for evidence of extraocular spread of the tumour and any associated complications such as cataract, corneal oedema from secondary glaucoma or subluxation of the lens.

References

1. Hoh, H.B., Menage, M. and Dean-Hart, J.C. (1993) Iris cyst after traumatic implantation of an eyelash into the anterior chamber. *British Journal of Ophthalmology*, **77**, 741–2
2. Shields, J.A and Shields, C.L. (1992) *Intraocular Tumours: a Text and Atlas*. W.B. Saunders, Philadelphia, pp. 61–84

Hyperoleon

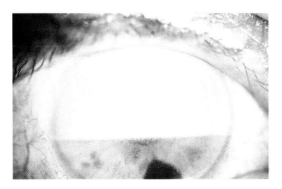

There is a fine suspension of silicone globules which has emulsified to form a 'hyperoleon' in the anterior chamber. Silicone oil is a polymer with varying lengths of siloxane (combination of silica and oxygen) units which account for the high viscosity of the liquid with a specific gravity of 1.9.

Intravitreal silicone oil is used as internal tamponade in a variety of vitreoretinal procedures.[1]

- Dissection of epiretinal membranes and flattening of the retina.
- Closure of breaks (especially inferior ones) which are complicated by PVR or PDR.
- Giant retinal tears.
- Complex or traumatic retinal detachments.

There are distinct advantages and disadvantages of silicone oil over gases. The advantages are that they:

- Are long-acting.
- Maintain a constant size of globule and refractive index which allows fundal visualization.

The disadvantages are that they induce:[2]

- Cataract formation.
- Pupillary-block glaucoma in the aphakic eye (which can be prevented with the Ando iridectomy at 6 o'clock) and secondary open angle glaucoma (due to trabecular blockage by silicone globules).
- Keratopathy.
- Possible retinal and optic nerve toxicity.

Management

The emulsified silicone oil should be removed.

References

1.   Leaver, P.K. (1992) Use of intravitreal liquid silicone. New approaches to vitreoretinal surgery. *International Ophthalmology Clinics*, **32** (2), 81–93
2.   Federman, J.L. and Schubert, H.D. (1988) Complications associated with the use of silicone oil in 150 eyes after retina-vitreous surgery. *Ophthalmology*, **95**, 870–6

Endophthalmitis

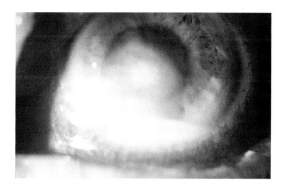

There is pus in the anterior chamber with a 3 mm fluid level (hypopyon) just below the pupil in an eye which has a penetrating keratoplasty. Other signs include conjunctival hyperaemia, flare and cells in the anterior chamber. This is consistent with a postoperative endophthalmitis which has an incidence of approximately 0.1%.[1]

Differential diagnosis

Includes a sterile hypopyon associated with a chronic uveitis secondary to an autoimmune cause such as a connective tissue disease like sarcoidosis or ankylosing spondylitis. Risk factors for postoperative endophthalmitis include:

- Preoperative ocular risks include diabetics, patients with poor tear film, keratoconjunctivitis sicca, blepharitis or infective conjunctivitis.
- Perioperative risks such as inadequate instrument sterilization and long intraocular instrumentation time, broken posterior capsule, i.e. use of intraocular lens with prolene haptics.
- Postoperative immunosuppression (steroids etc.) or leakage from the surgical section.

Investigations

Investigations revolve around the identification of the organism through microscopy, staining (Gram, Giemsa, Gomori's silver stain) and culture of the sample derived from:

(a) Swabbing of the surface ocular structures like the conjunctiva.
(b) Anterior chamber tap or vitreous biopsy (via needle aspiration or pars plana vitrectomy).
(c) Ultrasound or CT scan to exclude the presence of intraocular foreign body.

Diagnostic cultures are performed on standard agar plates such as chocolate agar which identifies Neisseria and Haemophilus, Sabourand's agar (identifies fungi) and blood agar which differentiates haemolytic bacteria from non-haemolytic species.

Management

The principle of treatment relies on prompt diagnosis and is aimed at eradicating the offending organism.

1. Medical
    * Antibiotics, topical, systemic or intravitreal.
    * Topical steroids to reduce inflammation are usually given when the infection has been brought under control.
2. Surgical intervention with a therapeutic vitrectomy to reduce infective organism load.
3. Infection control should be notified if there is a sudden outbreak of cases arising from the operating theatres or wards.

Prognosis

Gram-negative endophthalmitis have a poor prognosis compared to infections caused by *Streptococcus epidermidis* or *Propionibacterium acnes*.

Reference

1. Bauman, W.C. and D'Amico, D.J. (1992) Surgical techniques in diagnosis and management of suspected endophthalmitis. New approaches to vitreoretinal surgery. *International Ophthalmic Clinics*, **32** (2), 81–93

Subluxated lens

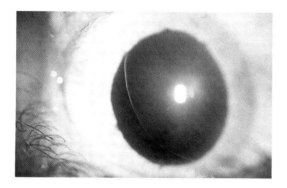

There is an upward and temporal subluxation of the lens in this eye. It remains in the posterior chamber and does not appear to be dislocated (i.e. completely detached from the zonules compared to partially detached in subluxation). There is no leakage of lens matter and the iris does not appear to be pushed forwards causing shallowing of the anterior chamber. This is consistent with a subluxated lens or ectopia lentis which is associated with inherited disorders such as homocysteinuria, aniridia, buphthalmos, Marfan's and Weill–Marchesani syndromes and secondary to acquired disorders like high myopia and hypermature cataract. In addition, uveitis due to syphilis, intraocular tumours and trauma may cause the lens to sublux or dislocate.

Investigations

The patient should be examined systematically and investigated to exclude systemic causes of ectopia lentis. Patients with homocystinuria may improve with a low cysteine or methionine diet and pyridoxine while Marfan's patients can have cardiac anomalies such as an ascending aortic aneurysm or valvular prolapse.

The eye should be examined carefully for other signs of trauma such as iridodialysis and choroidal rupture as this may be a very likely diagnosis. The intraocular pressure should be measured to exclude secondary glaucoma as a complication.

Management[1,2]

A subluxed lens which is not causing problems can be left alone. However, if it is associated with secondary problems of secondary glaucoma (either open or narrow angle glaucoma), lens-induced uveitis or visual disturbance due to glare from the edge effect of the lens or decentration of the lens, the lens should then be removed.

1.   The surgical technique depends on the location of the lens within the eye. Those located in the posterior chamber can be removed either as an intracapsular technique with a cryoprobe or via a lensectomy with an anterior vitrectomy if the vitreous face is disturbed. A posteriorly dislocated lens will need a pars plana total vitrectomy. The lens can either be aspirated with a vitreous cutter or floated up with heavy fluids.

2.   Implantation of an intraocular lens (IOL) is tricky due to the absence of the posterior capsule. Posterior chamber IOL will require fixation with either scleral or iris fixation sutures while anterior chamber IOL may also be an option if there is no risk of glaucoma due to angle problems in traumatic cases or Marfan's. The patient may be left aphakic with optical correction with a contact lens.

Prognosis

There is an increased risk of postoperative cystoid macular oedema.

References

1.   Plager, D.A., Parks, M.M., Helveston, E.M. and Ellis, F.D. (1992) Surgical treatment of subluxated lenses in children. *Ophthalmology*, **99**, 1018–23
2.   Hakin, K.N., Jacobs, M., Rosen, P. *et al.* (1992) Management of the subluxed crystalline lens. *Ophthalmology*, **99**, 542–5

Essential iris atrophy

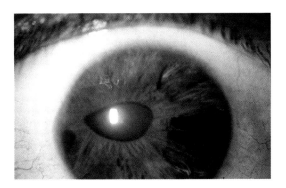

There is iris stromal atrophy with full-thickness iris hole formation at the 3 and 9 o'clock positions. In addition there is displacement of the pupil towards an area of peripheral anterior synechiae at the 9 o'clock position. This is characteristic of essential iris atrophy which is one of three clinical manifestations of a disease process known as iridocorneal endothelial (or ICE) syndrome. The other two include iris naevus or Cogan–Reese syndrome (characterized by diffuse iris naevus) and Chandler's syndrome which falls between the previous two entities. The disease is unilateral and typically occurs in women between the ages of 20 and 40 years with no inheritance pattern. Pathologically, there is an overgrowth of endothelial cells known as ICE-cells in the anterior chamber and trabecular meshwork with the formation of peripheral anterior synechiae resulting in raised intraocular pressure. Other signs include fine dark guttate-like lesions on the endothelium which gives the 'hammered' appearance and corneal oedema.

Differential diagnosis

Includes posterior polymorphous dystrophy (or PPD).

Investigations

(a)   Measurement of the intraocular pressure and gonioscopy to assess the extent of the peripheral anterior synechiae.
(b)   The morphology of the ICE cells can be appreciated under high magnification or using specular microscopy. In contrast, the endothelium has vesicles, bands and ridges in PPD.

Management

In the absence of secondary problems such as glaucoma, no treatment is required in ICE syndrome. However, these patients should be followed up regularly to detect evidence of raised intraocular pressure. Treatment is the same as open angle glaucoma, although the outlook is not so good.

Prognosis

All patients will eventually develop glaucoma.

Dense cataract

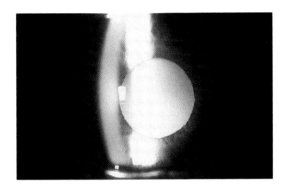

There is dense white cataract in this eye. This is consistent with a mature cataract which can be due to a variety of acquired causes such as age, trauma, radiation, inflammatory (chronic uveitis), drug-induced (such as steroids) and associated systemic diseases such as dystonic myotonia. Congenital causes include dominant inherited cataracts, intrauterine diseases such as rubella and trauma. The patient will experience symptoms of decreased visual acuity, glare, monocular diplopia and index myopia. Complications arising from a mature cataract include spontaneous dislocation, phacomorphic and phacolytic glaucoma.

Investigations

(a) An accurate ocular history usually determines the cause. The eye should be examined thoroughly to exclude other signs of trauma and uveitis.

(b) As a fundal view is difficult, a B-scan ultrasound is essential to ensure that there is no coexisting retinal problem such as a long-standing retinal detachment. Look for RAPD.

(c) Keratometry and axial lengths should be measured so that a suitable intraocular lens may be selected for implantation. It is essential that the patient's refraction (especially of the fellow eye) be known to ensure that the patient is not rendered anisometropic postoperatively. For example, making a high myope (-6 dioptres) emmetropic in the eye with a cataract will cause anisometropia.

(d) The macula should be examined so that the visual outcome may be predicted and the patient will not be unduly disappointed postoperatively.

Management

Indications for cataract extraction vary between different practitioners and hospitals. For example, some patients with visual acuity of 6/12 may be incapacitated by symptoms of glare. The treatment of a cataract is the surgical removal and an intraocular lens (IOL) implantation.

1. Removal of a cataract is surgical and can be:
    - Intracapsular extraction, which is now reserved for a dislocated lens.
    - Extracapsular extraction.
    - Phacoemulsification.
2. Implantation of an intraocular lens (IOL) can either be in the anterior or more commonly in the posterior chamber. The only contraindication to IOL implantation is pre-existing ocular inflammation. Loss of the posterior capsule is no longer an indication for anterior chamber IOL as posterior chamber IOL can be fixated on the iris or the sclera.
3. Postoperatively, the patient should have topical antibiotics as prophylaxis and topical steroids to reduce postoperative inflammation in the first 2 weeks.
4. At around 2 months postoperatively, the patient should be refracted and appropriate spectacle correction prescribed.

Keratic precipitates

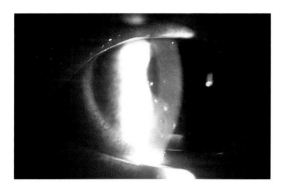

This is a slit-lamp view demonstrating keratic precipitates (inflammatory cellular infiltrates) on the endothelial surface of the inferior cornea. This is suggestive of uveitis (inflammation of the uveal tract) which can be classified as anterior (or iritis), intermediate (or pars planitis) or posterior uveitis and can be either active or chronic. Signs of active anterior uveitis include limbal hyperaemia (or ciliary flush), cells in the anterior chamber and aqueous flare, while chronic disease is associated with posterior synechiae, iris atrophy, iris nodules and secondary cataract formation.

Aetiology includes (i) idiopathic; (ii) exogenous causes such as penetrating injury or infectious agents (toxoplasmosis, toxocariasis, tuberculosis and leprosy); and (iii) endogenous causes such as seronegative arthritis (ankylosing spondylitis, psoriasis, Reiter's syndrome, juvenile chronic arthritis), sarcoidosis, Behcet's disease, Fuch's heterochromic cyclitis and sympathetic uveitis.

Investigations

(a) An accurate history will exclude penetrating injury as a cause. Careful ocular examination is required to assess the severity of the inflammation and determine whether the uveitis is confined to the anterior segment or if the posterior segment is involved.

(b) A full blood count, autoimmune profile and viscosity can pick up chronic systemic diseases.

(c) A chest X-ray may be abnormal in sarcoidosis, systemic lupus erythematosus or tuberculosis.

(d) Diagnostic tests such as a Kveim, Mantoux or HLA testing may be useful.

Management

1. An infectious cause should be eliminated with the appropriate treatment.

2. Active inflammation should be treated with immunosuppression such as steroids or steroid-sparing agents such as cyclosporin and azathioprine. Topical treatment may be sufficient for mild inflammatory process but severe reaction or posterior uveitis usually requires systemic treatment. It is important to manage uveitis early and aggressively to prevent secondary complications such as posterior synechiae, cataract formation, band keratopathy, rubeosis, secondary glaucoma, retinal detachment or phthsis bulbi.
3. Topical mydriatics should be given to prevent formation of posterior synechiae and to keep the eye comfortable.

Anterior fluorescein angiography

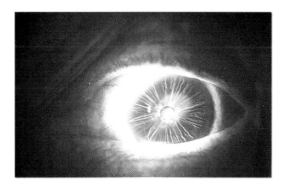

This is an anterior fluorescein angiography demonstrating normal iris vasculature in a radiating wheel-spoke like appearance. Although rarely performed, this test can be used to detect the following abnormalities:

- Anterior segment ischaemia, which can be consequent to alkali burns, multiple muscle strabismus surgery and retinal detachment surgery.
- Iris vessel anomalies such as capillary haemangiomas.
- Iris tumours.

Macula

Diabetic maculopathy

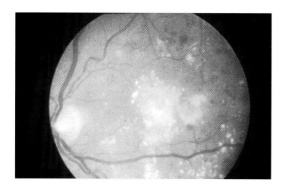

There is a circinate ring of yellowish hard exudates at the macula encroaching the fovea which appears to be oedematous. In addition, the macula shows presence of microaneurysms but absence of haemorrhages, cotton-wool spot or telangiectasis. This suggests a diagnosis of exudative diabetic maculopathy (DM), more commonly found in type 2 diabetes mellitus and one of the commonest causes of visual impairment in diabetes. There are two forms of diabetic maculopathies; the exudative and the ischaemic maculopathy.[1]

Differential diagnosis

Includes exudates arising from a macroaneurysm, congenital retinal telangiectasis (Coats' syndrome) and acquired juxtafoveolar retinal telangiectasis.

Investigations

(a) Full fundal examination should be carried out to detect other diabetic changes.
(b) Fluorescein angiography is not necessary as the diagnosis is a clinical one. It can detect the vascular abnormalities described above such as microaneurysmal changes in the capillary bed, the source of exudative leakage and macular oedema.[2] Clinically significant macular oedema is defined as either retinal oedema (or exudates) within 500 µm of the fovea or oedema 1500 µm in diameter within 1500 µm of the fovea.[3] Ischaemic changes can be recognized by areas of capillary non-perfusion in the macula and implies a poor prognosis.

Management

Exudative DM is a serious condition which needs early intervention before irreversible damage sets in. Treatment does not help in ischaemic DM.

1.   It requires prompt referral for treatment of focal argon laser burns of around 50–100 μm applied for 0.1 sec at the sites of leakage but ensuring the fovea is spared. The patient is reviewed at around 6–8 weeks to ensure resolution of both oedema and exudates.
2.   Prior to discharge the patient should be advised to present to the ophthalmic practitioner should symptoms of visual loss or meta-morphopsia occur.

Prognosis

Poor prognostic indicators include macular oedema, diffuse leakage and capillary non-perfusion at the macula. Patients with co-existing systemic diseases such as hypertension and renal failure also tend to have a poor outcome.

Tips

Also look for evidence of other ocular changes in diabetes such as prolif-erative disease (new vessels at the disc (NVD) or elsewhere (NVE) and rubeosis irides) and cataracts.

References

1.   Whitelocke R.A.F., Kearns, M., Blach, R.K. (1979) The diabetic maculopathies. *Transactions of the Ophthalmology Society*, **99**, 314–20
2.   Gass, J.D.M. (1987) *Stereoscopic Atlas of Macular Diseases: Diagnosis and Treatment, 3rd edn*, Mosby, St Louis, pp. 333–454
3.   Early Treatment Diabetic Retinopathy Study Group (1991) *Ophthalmology* (Suppl. 5), **98**, 739–834

Cystoid macular oedema

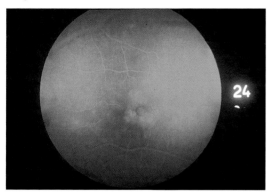

This is a fluorescein angiogram of a right eye at late venous phase showing perifoveal dye leakage in a petalloid pattern (representing dye leaked into the cystoid spaces in the outer retinal plexiform layer of Henle) more clearly seen in the picture taken 1 hour after the injection. This is consistent with cystoid macular oedema (CMO) and can be detected in 5–15% of patients following normal uncomplicated cataract extraction and especially if there was vitreous loss (Irving–Gass syndrome).

Other causes include oedema found in:

- Idiopathic cases.
- Retinal vascular disorders (retinal vein occlusion, diabetic maculopathy, vasculitis, telangectasia).
- Toxicity such as topical adrenaline in aphakics.
- Retinitis pigmentosa, X-linked juvenile retinoschisis.
- Chronic uveitis of any cause.
- Other intraocular procedures (penetrating keratoplasty, laser treatment such as argon PRP or YAG capsulotomy).

Investigations

Investigations should be directed at the cause of CMO.

Management

Treat the condition early to prevent permanent damage secondary to prolonged oedema or the development of a lamellar (pseudo-hole) macular hole which is irreversible to treatment.

1. Treat underlying condition (withdraw offending drug, treat uveitis etc.)
2. Systemic carbonic anhydrase inhibitors may be of value in treating surgery induced CMO.
3. Grid macular photocoagulation (between 50 and 150 low intensity 50 μm size spots) may dry the oedema caused by retinal vascular disease.

Macular hole

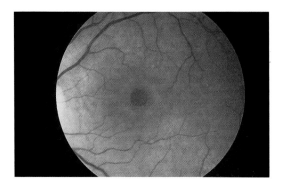

There is a round hole the size of 1/3 to 1/2 disc diameter in the centre of the macula, surrounded by a grey halo of retina detachment with yellow 'nodules' within the hole at the level of the retinal pigment epithelium. These features are consistent with a macular hole giving symptoms of central scotoma and metamorphopsia.

Causes of macular holes are:

* Idiopathic. It is thought that 70% arise in women, especially between the ages of 60 and 80 years, perhaps as a consequence of posterior vitreous detachment.
* Trauma.
* Solar retinopathy.
* High myopia.
* As consequence of traction from a peripheral epiretinal membrane.

Differential diagnosis

Includes a pseudomacular hole (a defect within an epiretinal membrane) or a lamellar hole secondary to chronic macular oedema.

Grading of macular hole[1]

Stage 1 Localized contraction of prefoveal cortical vitreous resulting in localized foveolar detachment from retinal pigment epithelium. A fluorescein angiogram (FFA) at this stage is normal. This may resolve spontaneously or progress to stage 2.

Stage 2 Early small full thickness defect (either in a crescentic or round shape) in the neuroretina between RPE and vitreous. The patient usually has visual loss due to the hole which can be seen in an FFA.

Stage 3 Full thickness hole with incomplete vitreous detachment.

Stage 4 Complete posterior vitreous separation resulting in an operculum (fragment of retina) suspended in front of the fovea.

Investigations

(a) Nil required as the diagnosis is a clinical one.

(b) Fluorescein angiogram may be useful as it shows up the full-thickness hole as a well-delineated zone of hyperfluorescence surrounded by a zone of less intense hyperfluorescence in the early (choroidal) phase and differentiates it from a pseudo- or lamellar hole, neither of which have this 'window defect' in FFA.

Management[2]

1. In established full-thickness holes, there is little one can do.

2. However, in impending hole formation, i.e. stages 2 or 3 (or if there is metamorphopsia in the fellow eye of an eye with a pre-existing hole), vitreous surgery with the removal of vitreous cortex to release tractional forces on the fovea with or without internal tamponade appears to prevent full-thickness hole formation.[3] However, this opinion is still controversial and a prospective multicentre randomized clinical trial is currently under way to resolve this issue.

Prognosis

Visual acuity is unlikely to be better than 6/60 in a full-thickness hole. The fellow eye has a 10% risk of developing the condition within 2 years. Following vitrectomy, 75% of successfully treated eyes improve by 2 or more lines of visual acuity due to the release of vitreous traction on the hole.

Tips

1. Assess the depth of the hole. There is a complete interruption of a fine slit beam focused over the hole (Watzke's sign).

2. Look for the operculum as evidence of posterior vitreous detachment.

3. There may be an epiretinal membrane in 10% of cases.

References

1. Gass, J.D.M. (1988) Idiopathic senile macular hole: its early stages and pathogenesis. *Archives of Ophthalmology*, **106**, 629–39

2. Sebag, J. (1992) Anatomy and pathology of the vitreo-retinal interface. *Eye*, **6**, 541–52

3. de Bustros, S. and Wendel, R.T. (1992) Vitrectomy for impending and full-thickness macular holes. New approaches to vitreoretinal surgery. *International Ophthalmic Clinics*, **32** (2), 81–93

Epiretinal membrane

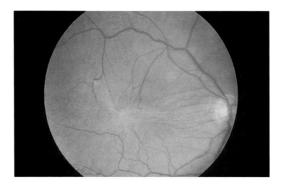

There appears to be puckering of the retina around the centre of the fovea with dragging of retinal vasculature towards this epicentre suggestive of an epiretinal membrane. Symptoms experienced by the patient would be metamorphopsia and blurring of vision.

Causes of epiretinal membrane are:

* Idiopathic (unilateral condition in the elderly, may be bilateral in 20%).
* Consequence of retinal vascular disorders (BRVO, CRVO, diabetes).
* Trauma.
* Chronic uveitis.
* Post-retinal detachment or following argon laser or cryotherapy of the retina.

Clinical diagnosis of a membrane is obvious although it may be mistaken for choroidal folds.

Investigations

(a) Fluorescein angiogram shows distortion of retinal vasculature around the epiretinal membrane. In addition, there may be cystoid macular oedema or leakage from perifoveal capillaries due to traction exerted.
(b) Exclude treatable cause.
(c) Accurate assessment of best corrected vision to detect deterioration early.

Management[1]

1. Treat underlying causes.
2. If membrane is stable and vision is not compromised, regular observations will be sufficient as the majority are non-progressive.

3. If there is severe visual impairment, intervention may be in the form of pars plana vitrectomy and membrane peel to relieve traction upon the retina.

Tips

1. The membrane and the retinal pucker is best seen with 'red-free' light in the early stages.
2. Look for a 'pseudo-hole'.

References

1. de Bustros, S., Thompson, J.T., Michels, R.G. *et al.* (1988) Vitrectomy for idiopathic epiretinal membranes causing macular pucker. *British Journal of Ophthalmology*, **72**, 692–5
2. Pesin, S.R., Olk, R.J., Grand, M.G. *et al.* (1991) Vitrectomy for pre-macular fibroplasia: prognostic factors, long-term follow-up, and time course of visual improvement. *Ophthalmology*, **98**, 1109–14

Age-related macular degeneration (ARMD)

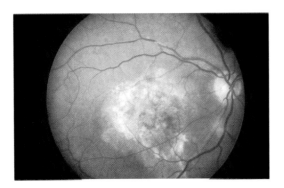

There is retinal pigment epithelium atrophy, pigment clumping and scar formation. This is consistent with age-related macular degeneration, a chronic degenerative disease affecting the choriocapillaris, Bruch's membrane and retinal pigment epithelium (RPE) thought to be consequent to deposition of lipid material (recognized clinically as drusen) within the Bruch's membrane. This phenomenon, which occurs with ageing, results in increasing hydrophobicity of the membrane. Other signs include subretinal neovascularization with exudates, (retinal) pigment epithelium detachment (PED), geographical choriocapillaris atrophy and an end-stage disciform scar.

ARMD can be divided into two main forms:

- 'Dry' ARMD, consisting mainly of drusen, pigment clumping and choriocapillaris atrophy.
- 'Wet' ARMD, which is characterized by the presence of subretinal neovascular membrane (SRNVM) and exudates (in addition to the features of 'dry' ARMD).

Differential diagnosis

Differential diagnosis of an ARMD scar includes an amelanotic choroidal melanoma or a disciform scar secondary to high myopia (Foster–Fuch's spot).

Investigations

(a) Nil required as this diagnosis is often clinically obvious. However, in doubtful cases or if SRNVM is suspected, a fluorescein angiogram (FFA) may be helpful.

(b) Fluorescein angiogram often reveals the following changes:

- Fluorescence at the early phase corresponding to the areas of drusen deposition with overlying RPE thinning or atrophy.
- Delayed choroidal perfusion.
- Presence of SRNVM can be detected by discrete areas of leakage which gradually enlarges with time (seen compared to a late FFA picture).
- PED shows up as a well-defined discrete area of fluorescein leakage which remains the same size throughout the period of angiography.
- Fluorescein staining of drusen.

Management

This depends on the stage of ARMD.[1]

1. In the 'dry' type with drusen and choriocapillaris atrophy only, no treatment is required. However, patients should be warned of symptoms of SRNVM such as deterioration of metamorphopsia and vision so that they may present early for treatment. The patient should be instructed on the use of an Amsler chart.
2. With the 'wet' type in the presence of SRNVM, using focal argon laser to obliterate areas of choroidal neovascularization which manifest as areas of leakage of FFA (provided the posterior edge of the lesion is 200 μm from the centre of the foveal avascular zone) at an early stage may prevent haemorrhages and subsequent development of a disciform scar. Successfully treated patients should be warned that they may lose 2–3 lines of visual acuity immediately after treatment, which remains stable thereafter.

The value of photocoagulation in PED is equivocal as this may increase the size of the detachment or cause the free edge of the epithelium to 'roll-under'. When a disciform scar has developed, there is no treatment available. However, counselling and advice on visual aids (such as magnifiers) at a low-visual aids clinic is of immense benefit in the visual rehabilitation of the patient. Registration as partially or fully blind may provide the patient with additional support.

Prognosis

The average age when visual loss occurs in the first eye is 65 years with a risk to the fellow eye of 5–10% annually.[2] Following a haemorrhage over the fovea from a SRNVM, 70% of patients will have vision less than 6/60.

References

1. Macular Photocoagulation Study Group. (1991) Subfoveal neovascular lesions in age-related macular degeneration. *Archives of Ophthalmology*, **109**, 1220–57
2. Gass, J.D.M. (1987) *Stereoscopic Atlas of Macular Diseases; Diagnosis and Treatment*, 3rd edn, Mosby, St Louis, pp. 60–97

Presumed ocular histoplasmosis syndrome (POHS)

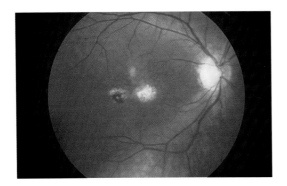

There are multiple well-circumscribed round yellowish nodules the size of 1/4 disc diameter at the macula. This is consistent with POHS due to a systemic infection with *Histoplasma capsulatum* which presents at about the age of 40 years. Other signs include punched-out atrophic scars of similar size and shape, peripapillary chorioretinal scarring and a band of depigmentation around the equator.

Differential diagnosis

- Pseudo POHS. (The patient is younger and there are smaller lesions which form clusters in quadrants. Unlike POHS which is asymptomatic unless the fovea is involved, these patients complain of floaters and photopsia).
- Multifocal choroiditis such as multiple toxoplasmosis or coccidioidomycosis.
- Punctate inner choroidopathy.
- Acute posterior multifocal placoid pigment epitheliopathy (APMPPE) which is self-limiting bilateral disease with characteristic punched-out lesions which block choroidal fluorescence in the early phase of the FFA.
- Multiple evanescent white dot syndrome (MEWDS) consists of 100–200 µm discrete white dots at the level of the RPE, often unilateral with some vitreous cells and vascular sheathing. The dots show early hyperfluorescence and late staining on FFA.
- Birdshot (vitiliginous) chorioretinitis is a bilateral disease of women between 50 and 70 years of age and associated with HLA-A29. There are vitreous cells and multifocal oval creamy-looking lesions with indistinct margins which result in visual loss and nyctalopia.

Investigations

(a) A positive skin reaction to subcutaneous injection of 1:1000 histoplasmin occurs in 90% of patients although only 16–68% of cases show presence of antibodies in the serum.
(b) A chest X-ray may reveal healed histoplasmosis.
(c) FFA may detect the presence of SRNVM with these lesions.

Management

Although there is no universal consensus, the following have been tried.

1. High dose systemic steroids (40–100 mg prednisolone daily) for those with a recent history of visual loss.
2. Argon photocoagulation to areas of SRNVM which lie more than 200 μm outside the centre of the foveal avascular zone (FAZ) reduces the risk of visual loss by three-fold.[1] If the lesion is between 1 and 199 μm from the FAZ (i.e. juxtafoveal), there is a 25% chance of the SRNVM still persisting after treatment.

Prognosis

Visual prognosis is related to the presence of SRNVM and its proximity to the fovea.[2] Patients with lesions outside the FAZ have a 60% chance of retaining 6/12 or better vision although this figure drops to below 15% if the lesion is within this zone. There is a risk of symptoms developing in the fellow eye in 22% of cases after 10 years.

References

1. Macular Photocoagulation Study Group. (1983) Argon laser photocoagulation for ocular histoplasmosis. *Archives of Ophthalmology*, **101**, 1347–57
2. Lewis, M.L., Van Newkirk, M.R. and Gass, J.D.M. (1980) Follow-up study of presumed ocular histoplasmosis syndrome. *Ophthalmology*, **87**, 390

Traumatic chorioretinal rupture (sclopetaria)

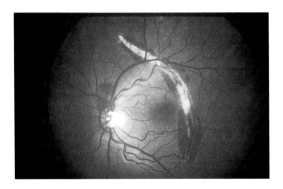

There is a vertical white streak in the posterior pole temporal to the fovea. This is consistent with a full-thickness break of the choroid and retina or chorioretinal rupture (sclopetaria) which separates to expose bare sclera underneath.[1] This is a rare manifestation of a blunt non-penetrating injury to the eye.

Investigations

(a) In view of previous trauma sustained, the eye should be examined for evidence of further damage such as:
  • Corneal decompensation and Descemet's splits.
  • Angle recession and accompanying raised IOP if there is more than 180° angle recession.
  • Post-traumatic mydriasis and iridodialysis.
  • Cataract and lens subluxation.
  • Posterior vitreous detachment and vitreous haemorrhage.
  • Retinal dialysis and retinal tears.
  • Relative or complete afferent reflex if there has been optic nerve contusion or damage.
(b) Fluorescein angiography is unnecessary. It will merely reveal the rupture as a dark streak with absent choroidal filling and normal overlying retinal vessels.

Management[2]

1. In the absence of a retinal detachment, tear or any other ocular damage, the eye should be left alone.
2. Any ocular complications arising from the initial injury should be treated. Secondary glaucoma should be treated as in primary OAG while retina tears or detachment should be repaired accordingly.

Greater care should be taken with the removal of a post-traumatic cataract due to weakening of the zonules which may increase the risk of vitreous loss.

Prognosis

The risk of a retinal detachment is rare due to the firm attachments of the edges of the split, which prevents fluid from getting into the subretinal space. Visual acuity is unaffected if the fovea is spared but may deteriorate at a later stage due to the development of pigmentary retinopathy or subretinal neovascular membrane.[3]

References

1. Dean-Hart, J.C. *et al.* (1980) Indirect choroidal tears at the posterior pole: a fluorescein angiographic and perimetric study. *British Journal of Ophthalmology*, **64**, 59–67
2. Martin, D.F. *et al.* (1994) Treatment and pathogenesis of traumatic chorioretinal rupture. *American Journal of Ophthalmology*, **117**, 190–200
3. Wood, M.W. and Richardson, J. (1990) Indirect choroidal ruptures: aetiological factors, patterns of ocular damage and final visual outcome. *British Journal of Ophthalmology*, **74**, 208–11

Dominant drusen (Doyne's honeycomb choroiditis)

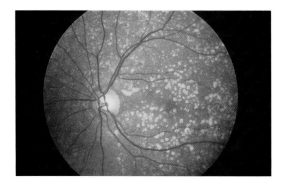

There are widespread discrete yellow lesions which look like drusen in the posterior pole. This is suggestive of dominant drusen or Doyne's honeycomb choroiditis which has an autosomal dominant inheritance pattern and is commonly seen in blue-eyed Caucasians.[1]

Differential diagnosis

Differential diagnosis of a 'flecked retina' at the posterior pole includes crystalline deposits due to tamoxifen, cystinosis or primary hereditary oxalosis and Alport's syndrome.

Drusen are focal collections of hyaline material deposited between the retinal pigment epithelium and Bruch's membrane and associated with local thickening of underlying Bruch's membrane, and atrophy of overlying retinal pigment epithelium. There are two distinct appearances – the 'soft' and 'hard' drusen – which may have prognostic implications.

Investigations

(a) Accurate assessment for other signs on the macula and peripheral retina in both eyes to exclude any other differential diagnosis. Stargardt's disease has flecks in the peripheral fundus and may be associated with a non-specific ('beaten-bronze') mottled appearance at the fovea.

(b) ERG is normal in familial dominant drusen but may be abnormal in Stargardt's disease due to RPE atrophy.

(c) Fluorescein angiography is useful if vision is affected and a subretinal neovascular membrane (SRNVM) is suspected.

Management

1. Having confirmed the diagnosis, the patient should be warned of a small risk of developing SRNVM which would require treatment. The patient should be advised to present to the clinician if symptoms of metamorphopsia develop and should therefore be issued with an Amsler chart for self-screening.
2. The development of an SRNVM requires treatment in the same manner as ARMD.

Prognosis

Due to the hydrophobic nature of 'soft' drusen, there appears to be an increased risk in developing SRNVM, while 'hard' drusen is associated with pigment epithelial detachment.

Reference

1. Gass, J.D.M. (1987) *Stereoscopic Atlas of Macular Diseases: Diagnosis and Treatment*, 3rd edn, Mosby, St Louis, pp. 60–5

Retina

Central retinal vein occlusion (CRVO)

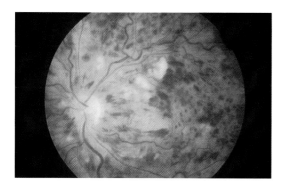

There is widespread retinal haemorrhage extending from a swollen optic disc involving all quadrants. Several cotton-wool spots (axonal material) are present superotemporally and the macula appears oedematous. Rubeotic vessels should be excluded from the iris/angle, IOP measured and pupillary reflexes tested to detect a relative afferent pupillary defect (RAPD). This is consistent with a haemorrhagic central retinal vein occlusion which is associated with the elderly, glaucoma, hyperviscosity states, hypertension and smoking.

Differential diagnosis

Although the diagnosis is usually clinically obvious, it may be mistaken for diabetic retinopathy.

Investigations

(a) Full blood count, viscosity to rule out hyperviscosity states such as myeloma.
(b) Blood pressure measured.
(c) Intraocular pressure measured and fellow disc assessed for evidence of glaucoma.
(d) Fluorescein angiography when haemorrhages clear (usually around 3–6 weeks) to look for ischaemia, especially if there are signs such as cotton-wool spots present.

Management

The principle lies in the prevention of the development of neovascularization and minimizing macular oedema.

1. Treat underlying systemic disease if present (the fellow eye is at risk of CRVO if the underlying disease remains untreated).

2.   Do nothing until after FFA.
3.   If FFA shows:
- No capillary closure, review regularly to ensure signs of ischaemia (cotton wool spots, new vessels at the disc and iris) do not occur. These occur usually around 3 months (hence the term '100-day rubeotic glaucoma') and need treatment, as below.
- Extensive capillary closure (or 'drop-out'), argon pan-retinal photocoagulation is required.[1]
- Macular oedema, grid macular photocoagulation (between 50 and 150 low intensity 50 μm size spots) will dry the macula.

Prognosis

Young patients have a good prognosis and may return to within 2 lines of vision. Poor prognostic factors include extensive capillary closure and presence of relative afferent pupillary defect. There is a 10% chance of CRVO occurring in the fellow eye.[2]

Reference

1.   Hayreh, S.S., Klugman, M.R., Podhajsky, P. *et al.* (1990) Argon laser panretinal photocoagulation in ischaemic central retinal vein occlusion. *Graefes Archives of Clinical Experimental Ophthalmology*, **228**, 281–96
2.   Pollack A., Dottan, S., and Oliver, M. (1989) The fellow eye in retinal vein occlusive disease. *Ophthalmology*, **96**, 842–5

Branch retinal vein occlusion (BRVO)

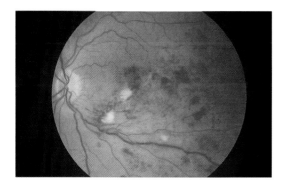

There is flame-shaped haemorrhage originating from the disc along the superotemporal quadrant with exudates present. There is no evidence of cotton-wool spots or new vessel formation or macula oedema. This is suggestive of branch retinal vein occlusion or BRVO and is associated with ageing and hypertension which results in the arteriole nipping the venule as they share the same adventitial sheath.[1]

Investigations

As for central retinal vein occlusion (CRVO).

Management

The principle lies in prevention of the complications, namely new vessel formation (NVE), and minimizing macular oedema.

1. Treat underlying systemic disease.
2. Do nothing until after FFA. This should be performed when the haemorrhages have cleared to detect areas of capillary non-perfusion.
3. If FFA shows:
   - No capillary closure at the involved quadrant, observe regularly for at least 3 years as NVE may develop. This is seen later than following CRVO and occurs usually around 6–12 months. If NVE occurs, treat with sectoral argon retinal photocoagulation.
   - Capillary closure at involved quadrant, sectoral argon retinal photocoagulation is required. If the closure involves more than 2 quadrants (i.e. hemivein occlusion), the treatment and prognosis is as CRVO.
   - Macula oedema, treatment with grid macular photocoagulation (between 50 and 150 low intensity 50 μm size spots) may dry the macula.

Prognosis

Inferior and nasal BRVOs have a better visual prognosis as the macula is not affected.

Reference

1.   The Eye Disease Case-Control Study Group (1993) Risk factors for branch vein occlusion. *American Journal of Ophthalmology*, **116**, 286–96

Central retinal arterial occlusion

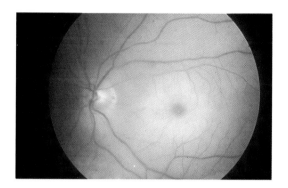

There is generalized pallor of the fundus and disc with marked narrowing of retinal arterioles. The orange reflex from the choroid remains at the fovea giving the 'cherry-red spot' sign. This is consistent with a central retinal arterial occlusion which can be caused by:[1]

- Emboli from the heart (diseased heart valves, thrombus following an infarct or rarely atrial myxoma) or from stenosed carotid arteries.
- Vaso-obliterative disorders such as atheroma (age-related) or vasculitides (giant cell arteritis or collagen vascular diseases).
- Excessive high intraocular pressure following acute angle closure glaucoma or retinal detachment surgery.

Differential diagnosis

The 'cherry-red spot' sign can also be seen in the fundus of a rare group of metabolic diseases known as sphingolipidoses.

Investigations

Investigations are directed at excluding treatable causes.

(a) General systemic examination (listen for carotid bruits and heart murmurs).
(b) Raised blood viscosity and ESR infers acute inflammation.
(c) Carotid doppler ultrasonography/arteriogram/subtraction angiography and cardiac imaging will detect flow abnormalities.
(d) Temporal artery biopsy provides definitive diagnosis in giant cell arteritis.

Management

Management is aimed at restoring the retinal circulation if the patient presents early (within 48 hours or so) and secondly at treating the underlying systemic condition.

1. The retinal perfusion can be increased by several methods aimed at dislodging the emboli.
    - Rebreathing into a paper bag causes hypercapnic induced vasodilatation.
    - Firm ocular massage.
    - Intravenous acetazolamide or anterior chamber paracentesis to induce sudden reduction of intraocular pressure.
2. Carotid artery stenosis or cardiac valvular abnormalities should be referred to cardiac and vascular surgeons for further management.
3. Vasculitides should be treated promptly with systemic immunosuppression.

Prognosis

The vision rarely improves beyond the visual acuity observed at presentation.

Tips

1. Look for a relative afferent pupillary reflex.
2. Auscultate for carotid bruits and heart murmurs.

Reference

1. Brown, G.C. and Magargal, L.E. (1982) Central retinal artery obstruction and visual acuity. *Ophthalmology*, **89**, 14–19

Retinitis pigmentosa

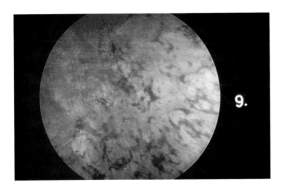

There are bone spicule pigmentary deposits in the mid-peripheral retina with attenuated retinal vessels and a pale, waxy optic nerve head.[1] Other signs include optic nerve drusen, posterior subcapsular lens opacity, maculopathy, open angle glaucoma and keratoconus. This is consistent with retinitis pigmentosa which can occur on its own or in association with other systemic diseases such as Usher's, Cockayne's, Kearn–Sayre, Laurence–Moon–Biedl and Bassen–Kornzweig syndromes. It affects 1 in 3000 people.

Most cases of RP are hereditary:[2]

- Autosomal dominant.
- Autosomal recessive.
- X-linked recessive.

A small number have an undetermined inheritance pattern.

Investigations

(a) Goldmann fields are constricted bilaterally.
(b) ERG shows a decreased amplitude in both scotopic and photopic b-wave. There is a delay between the flash of light and peak of b-wave as well as elevation of rod and cone thresholds in dark adaptation.
(c) EOG shows an absence of the light rise.

Management

1. Exclude and treat associated systemic diseases.
2. Genetic counselling.
3. Blind registration and low visual aids assessment where appropriate.
4. Recent studies have found that supplemental vitamin A (15,000 IU daily) appears to retard ERG changes in RP.

Prognosis

The patient initially suffers night blindness and progressive field loss. However, the central vision is later lost, typically by middle age, due to maculopathy and macula oedema for which there is no cure. The autosomal recessive type is most severe while patients with the autosomal dominant form may continue to have useful vision after the age of 40 years.

References

1. Dryja, T.P. (1992) Doyne Lecture. Rhodopsin and autosomal dominant retinitis pigmentosa. *Eye*, **6**, 1–10
2. Carr, R.E. and Noble, K.G. (1981) Disorders of the fundus: retinitis pigmentosa. *Ophthalmology*, **89**, 169–72

CMV retinitis

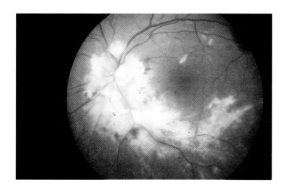

There is an arc-like geographical, swollen, yellow-white area with scattered haemorrhages (giving the 'pizza-like' appearance) along the inferotemporal arcade representing retinal necrosis and vasculitis. This is consistent with cytomegalovirus retinitis, an opportunistic infection associated with one-third of patients with HIV, haematological malignancies (lymphoma, leukaemia) and patients on immunosuppressive therapy. Other signs include conjunctival haemorrhages, quiet vitreous and slight anterior chamber flare.

Differential diagnosis

Differential diagnosis of infective retinitis are toxoplasmosis, toxocara, syphilis, tuberculosis, candida, acute retinal necrosis, cryptococcus and *Mycobacterium avium*.

Investigations

(a) Thorough personal (age, ethnic origin, environmental exposure, sexual behaviour) and medical histories (diabetes, immunosuppressive therapy).
(b) In addition to an ocular examination, there should be a general systemic examination.
(c) A full blood count detects evidence of haematological malignancies and immunosuppression. Serological tests for antibodies differentiate between an old (IgG) and newly acquired infection (IgM).
(d) Cultures for infectious agents should be performed on sputum (TB), blood (bacterial septicaemia) and vitreous if the diagnosis is not clinically obvious. Polymerase chain reaction (PCR) may be able to detect DNA of viral agents in question.

Management[1]

If possible, the patient's immune status should be returned to normal while anti-viral preparation is administered. However, due to the toxic side-effects of the virostatic agents gancyclovir (myelosuppression) and foscanet (renal toxicity), treatment should be given with caution. During treatment, the condition should be monitored with serial fundal photographs while white cell count and renal function are assessed for drug toxicity.

Indications of treatment are:

- Sight-threatening lesions.
- Large lesion measuring 4 disc diameters or more.
- Systemically symptomatic CMV illness.

More controversial are small peripheral lesions which have a slower rate of spread, and advanced disease which has rendered the eye blind.

Both gancyclovir and foscanet have to be given intravenously, usually through an indwelling Hickman line. The induction doses are 10 mg/kg and 200 mg/kg, whilst the maintenance doses are 5 mg/kg and 100 mg/kg for gancyclovir and foscanet respectively. However, even after resolution, maintenance treatment may still be required to prevent recurrences.

Prognosis

Resolution is seen in 60–80% of patients within 2 weeks of starting treatment, with peripheral lesions having a better prognosis due to slower growth. Blindness is due to sequential optic neuropathy, direct optic nerve involvement, retinitis at the macula and retinal detachment. Reactivation may occur in 30–50% of patients either at the junction of normal and diseased retina or as new lesions.

Reference

1.   Park, S.S. and D'Amico, D.J. (1992) Advances in antiviral therapy for cytomegalovirus retinitis. *Seminars in Ophthalmology*, **8**, 24–32

Toxoplasmosis

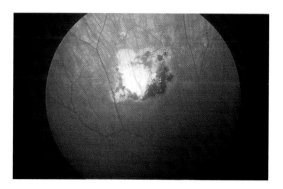

There is a focal oedematous narcotizing retinochoroiditis with indistinct edges at the macular region with overlying vitreous flare and cells at the edge of a pigmented scar. This is consistent with reactivation of toxoplasmosis (satellite lesion) at the site of a previous infection with the obligate intracellular protozon *Toxoplasma gondii.* The majority of ocular toxoplasmosis results from reactivation of latent retinal infection, either from transplacental congenital spread or more rarely from acquired infection through ingestion of food contaminated by cat faeces containing oocysts.[1]

Differential diagnosis

Includes toxocara, candida retinitis, acute retinal necrosis, syphilitic chorioretinitis and cytomegalovirus retinitis.

Investigations

(a) A thorough perinatal and medical history of previous systemic infections may help pinpoint the causative agents.
(b) A Mantoux test, chest X-ray, VDRL and TPHA will exclude tuberculosis and syphilis.
(c) Increasing serum viral and antibody titres using indirect fluorescent antibody, agglutination and ELISA tests can help to confirm the diagnosis.

Management

A small peripheral lesion needs only regular observation as the disease is usually self-limiting in immunocompetent patients. However, a clinical trial found that patients who received treatment tended to have a smaller scar than the non-treatment group.

In view of the toxic side-effects, treatment should only be given if:

- There is peri-papillary involvement (Jensen's choroiditis).
- The macula is encroached.
- There is a severe vitreous reaction.
- The vision is threatened.
- The patient is immunosuppressed or on immunosuppression therapy.

1. Medical treatment involves the following drugs, either singly or in combination for 4 weeks.
   - Sulphadiazine 150 mg/kg/day in four divided doses. As a sulphonamide, its side-effects are renal stones and allergic reactions such as Stevens–Johnson syndrome.
   - Pyrimethamine 1 mg/kg per day. Being a folic acid antagonist, it causes thrombocytopenia and leucopenia. As such, 5–10 mg/day of folinic acid is also given.
   - Steroid 0.5 mg/kg per day. This should never be used on its own as it may result in a fulminant toxoplasma infection.[2]
2. Surgery in the form of pars plana vitrectomy may be required to clear vitreous opacity caused by the infection.

Prognosis

Small lesions may self-limit over a period of a few months without treatment, although there may be episodes of reactivation in the future. Loss of vision occurs when the fovea or optic nerve is involved or when there is the formation of subretinal neovascular membrane (SRNVM) causing cystoid macular oedema, vitreous haemorrhage, tractional retinal detachment or scar formation.

References

1. Pierce, E.A. and D'Amico, D.J. (1992) Ocular toxoplasmosis: pathogenesis, diagnosis and management. *Seminars in Ophthalmology*, **8**, 40–52
2. Sabates, R., Pruett, R.C. and Brickhurst, R.J. (1981) Fulminant ocular toxoplasmosis. *American Journal of Ophthalmology*, **92**, 497–503

Acute retinal necrosis

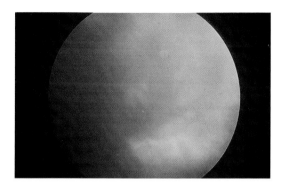

There is considerable vitreous flare and cells with confluent retinal necrosis in the periphery. This is consistent with acute retinal necrosis (ARN) thought to be associated with herpes zoster (following shingles or chicken pox), herpes simplex (following cold sores or encephalitis) and possibly Epstein–Barr viruses. Additional signs include anterior uveitis, optic neuritis and retinal detachment.[1]

Differential diagnosis

Includes toxoplasmosis, toxocara, candida and cytomegalovirus retinitis. These are usually more localized compared to the widespread lesions of ARN.

Investigations

(a) A thorough medical history of previous systemic infections may help pinpoint the causative agents.
(b) A Mantoux test and chest X-ray will exclude tuberculosis while VDRL and TPHA rules out syphilis.
(c) Increasing serum viral and antibody titres, with a positive culture from aqueous/vitreous tap or retinal biopsy, can be helpful.

Management

1. Systemic acyclovir reduces the risk of bilateral disease. It is given intravenously (10–15 mg/kg t.d.s.) for one week and then orally 800 mg five times daily for about one month.
2. The disease should be monitored regularly with serial fundal photography.

Prognosis

There is a risk of fellow eye involvement in one-third of cases.

Reference

1.   Sternberg, P., Hann, D.P., Yeo, J.H. (1988) Photocoagulation to prevent retinal detachment in acute retinal necrosis. *Ophthalmology*, **95**, 1389–93

Angioid streaks

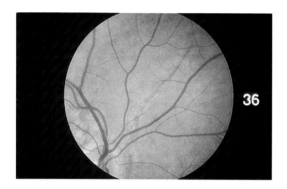

There are dark brown streaks with serrated edges radiating out from the optic disc. Other signs which can be seen are peripapillary atrophy, disciform scar, optic disc drusen, mid-peripheral retinal peau d'orange pigmentary mottling and crystalline bodies. These features are consistent with angioid streaks, which are linear dehiscence found in the collagenous and elastic portions of Bruch's membrane. Although 50% of the patients have no other systemic diseases, the other half may have the following conditions:[1]

- Pseudoxanthoma elasticum (Gronblad–Strandberg syndrome) in 85%.
- Ehlers–Danlos syndrome.
- Paget's disease (in 10%).
- Sickle-cell disease (in 1–2%).

Complications arising from the streaks which can result in loss of vision are choroidal SRNVM (which is seen usually after the fifth decade) and choroidal rupture following ocular trauma.

Investigations

(a) Exclude associated systemic diseases such as pseudoxanthoma elasticum.

(b) Fluorescein angiography (FFA) may be required to detect and locate a suspected SRNVM. In the early phase, FFA reveals the pattern of streaks as a 'window-defect' (due to atrophy of overlying retinal pigment epithelium) as a star around the optic disc. Complications such as SRNVM and choroidal rupture may manifest as areas of fluorescein leakage.

Management

1. The patient should be investigated medically to exclude the systemic diseases associated with angioid streaks. In particular, pseudoxanthoma

elasticum should be excluded as they may have hypertension, peripheral and coronary arterial disease which requires medical intervention. In addition genetic counselling should be offered for this autosomal recessive condition.

2. Angioid streaks do not need treatment. However, due to the brittleness of Bruch's membrane, patients should be warned of the high risk of choroidal rupture, and should therefore refrain from activities such as contact sports which may predispose to ocular trauma.

Reference

1. Gass, J.D.M. (1987) *Stereoscopic Atlas of Macular Diseases; Diagnosis and Treatment*, 3rd edn, Mosby, St Louis, pp. 102–9

Proliferative vitreoretinopathy (PVR)

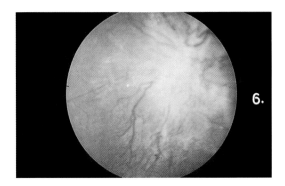

This is consistent with PVR stage C2 which is associated with post-retinal detachment surgery (the commonest cause of anatomical failure for rhegmatogenous retinal detachment surgery), retinal laser treatment, intraocular injection of silicone oil, following trauma, retinal vascular diseases and chronic intraocular inflammation.

There are two types of PVR – anterior and posterior – and both are due to fibrocellular (characterized by retinal pigment epithelium, fibrocyte and glial cells) proliferation resulting in traction on retina, ciliary body, iris and lens. Based on the extent of the membrane formation, PVR is divided into four stages:[1]

- Grade A – minimal PVR where there is hazy vitreous due to clumping of pigmented cells.
- Grade B – presence of wrinkling of inner retinal surface and vascular tortuosity.
- Grade C – presence of full-thickness, fixed retinal folds which is subdivided into:
  C1 – involvement of one quadrant of retina.
  C2 - involvement of two quadrants.
  C3 – involvement of three quadrants.
- Grade D – fixed retinal folds in all four quadrants and often associated with hypotony. This also subdivided into:
  D1 – wide funnel shaped folds.
  D2 – narrow funnel shaped folds.
  D3 – folds obscure the optic disc.

Management[2]

The surgical objective is to isolate retinal traction by separating the membrane from the retina, reattach any detached retina and ensure all retinal breaks are closed. Membrane peeling may be performed using the following techniques.

1.   Conventional scleral buckling may be useful in the early stages to prevent the establishment of fixed folds.
2.   Vitreoretinal surgery involving intravitreal membrane peeling combined with either gas or silicone is popular but has the disadvantage of leaving behind residual membrane.
3.   When PVR affects retina anterior to the ora serrata, retinal surgery involving retinotomy and retinectomy may be required to divide the peripheral retina in order to relieve traction at the macula.

Prognosis

Open funnel PVR with peripheral retinal involvement is more difficult to treat. PVR affecting retina anterior to the ora serrata has a poorer prognosis.

References

1.   Machemer, R., Aaberg, T.M., Freeman, H.M. *et al.* (1991) An updated classification of retinal detachment with proliferative vitreoretinopathy. *American Journal of Ophthalmology*, **112**, 159
2.   Aaberg, T.M. (1988) Management of anterior and posterior proliferative vitreoretinopathy. XLV Edward Jackson Memorial Lecture. *American Journal of Ophthalmology*, **106**, 519

Advanced proliferative diabetic retinopathy

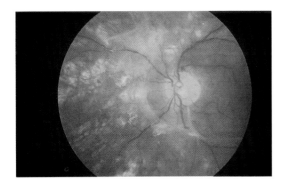

There is a tractional vitreoretinal membrane within the arterial arcades causing a small tractional retinal detachment (TRD). This is suggestive of an advanced diabetic retinopathy with tractional detachment.

TRD can be divided into:

- FTRD – any TRD with foveal detachment; or
- EFTRD – any TRD without foveal involvement, which can be within or outside of the major temporal vascular arcades.

This distinction is useful as patients with EFTRD may continue for an indefinite period with good visual acuity and foveal attachment, and as such may not need intervention.

Differential diagnosis

Includes proliferative vitreoretinopathy and epiretinal membrane.

Management

The appropriate management of tractional retinal detachment is complex although it is accepted that surgery should be deferred and the patient observed regularly unless the fovea or macula is involved or the membrane is progressing. Small membranes outside the macula region may be left. The risks of a vitrectomy should be balanced with the possible benefits received.

1. Although the timing of surgery is controversial, early vitrectomy to remove vitreous opacities and divide all tractional vitreoretinal membranes appears to be beneficial at 2 years of follow-up with 44% of patients maintaining a visual acuity of 6/12 or better.[1]
2. Photocoagulation to the retina should also be performed to reduce the risks of further neovascularization.

Prognosis

The incidence of visual loss in the diabetic population is 1.5–3%. This is associated with increasing duration of diabetes, severe retinopathy and presence of macular oedema.[2]

References

1. Diabetic Retinopathy Vitrectomy Study Research Group (1988) Early vitrectomy for severe proliferative diabetic retinopathy in eyes with useful vision. *Ophthalmology*, **95**, 1307–20
2. Moss, S.E., Klein, R. and Klein, B.E. (1988) The incidence of vision loss in a diabetic population. *Ophthalmology*, **95**, 1340–8

Proliferative diabetic retinopathy

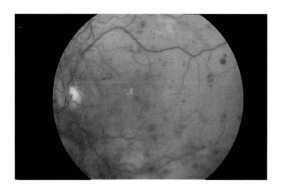

There are cotton-wool spots, blot haemorrhages, exudates, micro-aneurysms and new vessels at the peripheral retina. This is consistent with proliferative diabetic retinopathy. The pathology is a microangiopathy of the small vessels of the retina resulting in vessel leakage, haemorrhage and occlusion causing retinal ischaemia. In response to the ischaemia, growth factors are produced and these stimulate the production of new vessels which are unfortunately friable and bleed easily resulting in vitreous haemorrhages.[1]

Between 1 and 2% of the population have diabetes of which there are two types; namely the insulin (IDDM) and non-insulin dependent diabetes mellitus (NIDDM).

Investigations

(a) Fasting blood glucose confirms the diagnosis of diabetes which requires treatment.
(b) Diabetic retinopathy is a clinical diagnosis. Fluorescein angiography will merely confirm the presence of new vascularization at the disc (NVD) or elsewhere (NVE).

Management

Clinically, diabetic retinopathy can be divided into several stages according to the modified Airlie–House classification which dictates clinical management;

1. *Background* Microaneurysms with occasional exudates and 'dot' haemorrhages characterize this benign stage of retinopathy which is present in most diabetics after several years of developing diabetes. No action is required.
2. *Pre-proliferative* There are 'cotton-wool' spots, arteriolar narrowing, more exudates, 'larger blot' haemorrhages and intraretinal

microvascular anomalies (IRMA). This stage implies the presence of retinal ischaemia and will progress to the next stage in due course. Pan-retinal photocoagulation is required to reduce the areas of ischaemia.

3. *Proliferative* This stage is characterized by NVD and NVE which are prone to bleed causing vitreous haemorrhages. These patients warrant urgent pan-retinal photocoagulation as the vessels may regress if treatment is administered early.

4   *Advanced* This is the end-result of uncontrolled proliferative retinopathy resulting in vitreous haemorrhage and tractional retinal detachment. At this late stage, vitreoretinal surgery will be required to remove the blood clot and fibrovascular membrane formed within the vitreous to clear the visual axis.

Prognosis

Diabetic retinopathy is the commonest cause of blindness in the 30–60 years age group in the Western world. When there is NVD or NVE, there is a 40% and 7% chance of severe visual loss within 2 years respectively if they remain untreated. As such all diabetics should be screened and followed-up on a regular (half-yearly or yearly) basis for fundoscopy particularly when they have risk factors such as long duration of disease (10 years or more), smoking, hypertension or pregnancy. Diabetes affects not only the retina causing retinopathy but diabetics are more prone to developing cranial nerve palsies, cataracts, rubeotic glaucoma and ocular infections.

Reference

1. Ulbig, M.R. and Hamilton, A.M.P. (1993) Factors influencing the natural history of diabetic retinopathy. *Eye*, **7**, 242–9

Choroidal melanoma

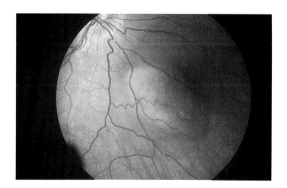

There is a pigmented, oval, well-demarcated and elevated lesion measuring 3 optic disc diameter (DD) just below the optic disc. This is consistent with a choroidal melanoma. Other signs which may point towards a melanoma are orange lipofuscin pigment lying on the tumour and exudative retinal detachment. Choroidal melanoma is the commonest primary intraocular tumour in adults (6 per 1 million) presenting at the age of 50 years, commonly found in male Caucasians and patients with oculodermal melanosis.

Differential diagnosis

Includes a choroidal naevus, age-related disciform scar, metastasis from skin melanoma, melanocytoma, retina pigment haematoma or hypertrophy.

Investigations

(a) Full ocular and systemic examination to detect extent of tumour spread.
(b) Indirect ophthalmoscopy to assess the diameter and elevation of the tumour as this affects management. Transillumination may help to differentiate a pigmented tumour (which does not transilluminate) from a exudative retinal detachment, choroidal detachment and non-pigmented tumours.
(c) A-scan ultrasonography shows an internal spike while B-scan demonstrates an acoustic hollowness, choroidal excavation and orbital shadowing behind the tumour.
(d) An MRI may be useful in delineating the extent of the tumour and its spread.
(e) Fluorescein angiography shows the lesion to be diffusely hyperfluorescent in the prearterial and arterial phases with a characteristic 'double circulation' of both choroidal and retinal vessels within the lesion.

(f)   Radioactive phosphate uptake test may be useful.
(g)   Ultrasound guided fine-needle aspiration is an option.
(h)   Liver function tests or liver ultrasound and chest X-ray to exclude systemic metastasis.

Management[1]

The management of the patient depends on a number of factors such as confirmation of the diagnosis, visual impact of the lesion, expected potential survival period and patient preference. The options are:

1.   In the case of doubtful diagnosis of a small lesion (less than 10 mm diameter and 2 mm height), regular monitoring with ultrasonography and photography will detect any growth.
2.   Enucleation is indicated if there is extensive involvement of the globe with extraocular spread, poor visual potential and presence of secondary glaucoma.
3.   Local resection is possible but technically difficult with a risk of retinal detachment.
4.   Charged particle irradiation using a collimated beam of protons or helium ions can be used if the lesion is 3 mm away from the optic disc. Complications include papillopathy and rubeotic glaucoma.
5.   Cobalt or iodine episcleral plaque radiation (brachytherapy) for anterior tumours less than 10 DD and 5 mm elevation.
6.   Low energy photocoagulation if the elevation is less than 5 mm. Photodynamic therapy which involves injection of photosensitizing dye such as haematoporphyrin and laser photocoagulation appears to be promising.

Prognosis

Poor prognostic factors include Callender epitheliod cell type (spindle A has a better prognosis than epitheliod cell type which has a 70% mortality at 5 years), large and diffuse tumours, pigmented tumours, extension beyond Bruch's membrane or sclera and distant metastasis. Factors associated with metastasis (mortality rate 87% after 1 year) are large tumour diameter, ciliary body involvement and older age of the patient at treatment. Interestingly, rapid initial tumour regression is also associated with a greater risk of metastasis, perhaps reflecting an initial faster rate of growth.[2]

References

1.   Damato, B.E. (1993) An approach to the management of patients with uveal melanoma. *Eye*, **7**, 388–97
2.   Augsburger, J.J., Gamel, J.W., Shields, J.A. *et al.* (1987) Post-irradiation regression of choroidal melanomas as a risk factor for death from metastatic disease. *Ophthalmology*, **94**, 1173–7

Choroidal haemangioma

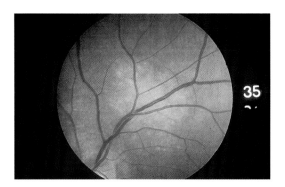

There is a circumscribed dome-shaped (placoid) red-orange lesion at the posterior pole with overlying mottling of the retinal pigment epithelium and yellow-white foci on the surface. This is consistent with a choroidal haemangioma although an amelanotic choroidal melanoma, choroidal osteoma, age-related macular degeneration or a metastatic tumour may mimic it. Other signs include metaplasia of retinal pigment epithelium into bone and exudative retinal detachment. Diffuse (not unifocal circum-scribed) haemangiomas may be associated with Sturge–Weber syndrome. This is the commonest vascular tumour of the choroid.

Investigations

(a) Imaging with A-scan ultrasonography shows a characteristic initial spike due to a high internal reflectivity. B-scan outlines the sharp border, internal acoustic solidity with no choroidal excavation in contrast to a choroidal melanoma.

(b) Fluorescein angiography shows the presence of irregular hyperfluo-rescence of large choroidal vessels in the early pre-arterial phase in the posterior pole. This can be better seen with indocyanine green angiography. Ninety-six per cent of choroidal haemangiomas are found in the posterior pole.

(c) Radioactive phosphate uptake test may be useful.

Management

In general, the tumours are asymptomatic and require no treatment. However, in the presence of serous retinal detachment, argon laser photo-coagulation may be required to create a choroidal–retinal adhesion and facilitate resolution of subretinal fluid.

Prognosis[1]

The lesion is benign and remains quiescent for years. If exudative retinal detachment occurs, the visual prognosis depends on the site of the lesion. Only 8% retained a vision of 6/9 in a subfoveolar haemangioma compared to 38% of those with an extramacular lesion.

Reference

1.   Shields, J.A. and Shields, C.L. (1992) *Intraocular Tumours: a Text and Atlas*, W.B. Saunders, Philadelphia, pp. 239–60

Retinoblastoma

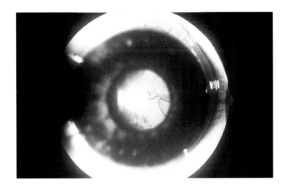

There is an absent red reflex or leucocoria in this child's eye with a manifest convergent strabismus. This is suggestive of a retinoblastoma.

Differential diagnosis

Conditions which may mimic retinoblastoma are as follows.

- Hereditary conditions such as Norrie's disease, incontinentia pigmenti, dominant exudative vitreoretinopathy and Coat's disease.
- Developmental abnormalities such as persistent hyperplastic primary vitreous (PHPV), retinopathy of prematurity, congenital cataract, retinal dysplasia, morning glory syndrome and myelinated fibres.
- Inflammatory disorders such as ocular toxocariasis and toxoplasmosis.
- Tumours such as choroidal haemangioma and retinal astrocytic haemartoma.
- Trauma causing vitreous haemorrhage or retinal detachment.

The commonest differential diagnoses are PHPV, Coat's disease and toxocariasis.

Investigations

(a) Ocular and systemic examination to exclude conditions mimicking retinoblastoma and detect signs of metastasis.
(b) Imaging of the tumour with ultrasound and CT can detect evidence of calcification while MRI gives a better soft tissue definition.
(c) Lumbar puncture to exclude metastasis in the central nervous system (CNS).

Management[1]

The main goals are the early removal of the tumour to decrease mortality by preventing local spread and metastasis, preservation of as much vision as possible, achievement of good cosmesis and genetic consultation. The therapeutic options, which depend on the size and location of the tumours, are as follows:

1. Enucleation is indicated if the tumour affects more than half the globe with extraocular extension, poor visual potential and presence of secondary glaucoma.
2. External beam radiotherapy (around 3500 rads in 9–20 fractions over a 4 week period) can be used as the tumours are radiosensitive. Indications include involvement of the maculo-papilla bundle, multiple tumours, vitreous seeding or tumours too large for cobalt plaque (more than 10 disc diameter or DD).
3. Cobalt episclera plaque radiation (brachytherapy) for anterior tumours less than 10 DD.
4. Cryotherapy (or photocoagulation) for tumours less than 3–4 DD and 2.5 mm elevation.

Prognosis

The overall mortality is around 5–15%. Poor prognostic factors are optic nerve and choroidal extension (where mortality increases to 50%), poor differentiation with absence of Flexner–Wintersteiner rosettes, and patients with hereditary retinoblastoma who are at risk of developing a second cancer at a later date. The tumour spreads by CNS extension via the optic nerve and haematogenous spread to bone, lymph nodes and liver via choroidal invasion.

Reference

1.   Mukai, S. (1993) Management of retinoblastoma. *Seminars in Ophthalmology*, **8**, 281–91

Intraocular metastasis

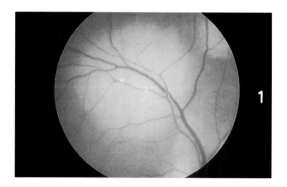

There is a creamy-yellow dome-shaped lesion with ill-defined borders in the posterior pole suggestive of a metastatic tumour most commonly from the breast or lung primary site. Other signs include mottled clumping of the retinal pigment epithelium and exudative retinal detachment.

Differential diagnosis

Includes amelanotic choroidal melanoma.

Investigations[1]

(a) Imaging with A-scan ultrasonography shows a moderate initial spike due to a high internal reflectivity while B-scan demonstrates internal acoustic solidity with no choroidal excavation unlike a choroidal melanoma.

(b) MRI imaging may be useful to differentiate between a metastatic lesion and a melanoma.

(c) Fluorescein angiography shows the lesion to be hypofluorescent in the early phase and diffusely hyperfluorescent in the late phase. There are no identifiable blood vessels within the lesion, unlike choroidal melanomas.

(d) Radioactive phosphate uptake test may be useful.

(e) Fine-needle aspiration is an option.

(f) Tests such as chest X-ray and mammogram will detect the primary lesion and liver function tests and ultrasound will demonstrate the extent of systemic metastasis.

Management

Although ocular metastasis is not a threat to the patient's survival, the management of the patient is complex and depends on a number of factors such as the extent of systemic spread, nature of primary disease, visual impact of the ocular lesion, expected potential survival period and patient preference. The options are:

1. External beam radiation or cobalt episclera plaque radiation (brachytherapy) may be useful if there is visual potential and the patient has a long survival period.
2. Chemotherapy.
3. Enucleation, especially if the eye becomes painful, rubeotic or phthisical.

Prognosis

The survival of the patient depends on the extent of systemic spread of the primary tumour at the time of diagnosis of ocular metastasis. Median survival period ranges from 3 months for skin melanomas, 5 months for lung cancer to 1 year for breast cancer as a primary site.

Reference

1. Augsburger, J.J. (1993) Intraocular metastatic tumours. *Seminars in Ophthalmology*, **8**, 241–7

Rhegmatogenous retinal detachment

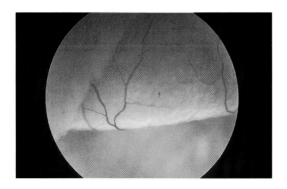

There is a fold of oedematous retina with underlying subretinal fluid (SRF) suggestive of a superior bullous rhegmatogenous retinal detachment (RD) arising from a break (either from a hole or tear) in the retina. Predisposing factors are pre-existing retinal degeneration (such as lattice degeneration, 'white without pressure', retinoschisis, snail-track degeneration and chorioretinal atrophy), high myopia, intracapsular extraction and post-YAG laser capsulotomy.

Signs of a fresh RD include a lowering of intraocular pressure (IOP), posterior vitreous detachment, vitreous haemorrhage and 'tobacco-dust' in the anterior vitreous while old RD develop subretinal demarcation lines at the junction of flat and detached retina, proliferative vitreoretinopathy, secondary intraretinal cysts, cataract formation and rubeosis. Most (60%) RD are due to a break in the superotemporal region although half the eyes have an additional break, usually located within one quadrant of each other.

Investigations

(a)   There is usually a history of floaters and photopsia.

(b)   Slit-lamp examination can detect lowering of the IOP and 'tobacco-dust'.

(c)   Indirect ophthalmoscopy and indentation is required to locate the site and extent of the tear to plan surgery. As SRF spreads in gravitational manner, the location of the tear can be found from the shape of the RD (Lincoff's principles); an inferior RD with equal fluid levels is due to a break at 6 o'clock while one with unequal levels will have a break at the side with the higher level. A superior-temporal RD is usually bullous with the SRF tracking inferiorly and around the optic disc to affect the nasal side. The fellow eye should be examined as 10% of RD are bilateral.

(d)   Ultrasonography may identify an RD if the fundal view is obscured by haemorrhage or cataract.

Management

This is an ophthalmic emergency and requires prompt intervention as the retina may become ischaemic within 48–72 hours. Prior to surgery, the patient's head should be positioned with the break lying inferiorly so that the SRF does not extend the RD any further. The type of surgery depends on the extent, numbers and sites of the tears. The considerations include the method of adhesion (argon laser or cryotherapy), scleral buckle (radial or circumferential), drainage of SRF, internal tamponade (air, SF6 or perfluorocarbon liquids) and vitreous surgery.

1. Cryotherapy of the break and scleral buckling using a silicone explant may be sufficient for a mobile RD with single posterior break and little SRF. A radial explant is sufficient for a single break while an encirclement is required for multiple (in more than one quadrant), anterior or wide breaks.
2. Drainage, air, cryotherapy and explant (DACE) is required for a highly elevated bullous RD. Instead of intravitreal air (which absorbs within 3–4 days), SF6 may be used instead as this will give internal tamponade for twice as long.
3. Pars plana vitrectomy may be required if there is PVR, dense vitreous haemorrhage or a giant tear extending more than two quadrants.

Panretinal photocoagulation of diabetic retinopathy

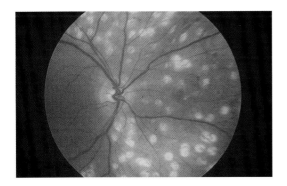

There are multiple white round areas of laser burns in the peripheral retina suggestive of a panretinal photocoagulation (PRP) for either proliferative diabetic retinopathy or ischaemic central retinal vein occlusion. These laser burns are old as there is pigment present at the edges of each burn. There is no evidence of new vessels or cotton-wool spots, which suggests that the treatment has been successful.

The mechanism by which PRP induces resolution of retinal neovascularization is unknown but two theories exist; the first that photocoagulation reduces the amount of vasoproliferative substance production while the second suggests that there is a greater diffusion of oxygen from the choroid to the inner retina following the destruction of the retinal pigment epithelium and outer retina.

Complications of retinal photocoagulation include:

- Early ones such as temporary decrease in visual acuity following laser, retrobulbar pain, haemorrhage, accidental photocoagulation of the fovea, acute retinal tear, cystoid macular oedema, macular and retinal holes, uveal effusion and field defects arising from loss of photoreceptors or nerve fibre layer within the burn area.
- Late complications, such as choroidal neovascularization, epiretinal membrane formation and contracture of an extensive burn causing retinal folds.

Tips

The fellow eye should be examined. Diabetes affects the fundus in both eyes while central retinal vein occlusion is usually unilateral.

Retinal vasculitis

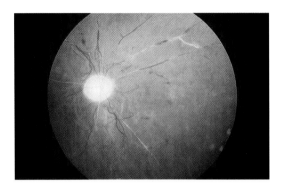

There is sheathing of the retinal arterioles with clear vitreous media suggesting the absence of vitritis. This is suggestive of retinal vasculitis which is defined as inflammation involving retinal vessels. Other signs include cotton-wool spots, retinal oedema and disc swelling. It is often associated with systemic diseases such as:

- Polyarteritis nodosa, Wegener's granulomatosis, systemic lupus erythematosus (SLE), sarcoidosis, Behçet's disease, multiple sclerosis and occasionally in seronegative arthropathies such as ankylosing spondylitis and Crohn's disease.
- Malignancy.

Investigations

(a) A careful ocular (patient usually complains of painless visual loss and floaters) and systemic history. There may be symptoms of associated systemic disease such as arthralgia, malaise and weight loss.

(b) Ocular examination of the posterior segment is important. There should be an absence of inflammatory cells in the vitreous. The type of vessel involvement may help in the diagnosis; inflammation involving the venules is more commonly seen in sarcoidosis and Behçet's disease.

(c) Haematological findings include chronic anaemia and increased blood viscosity. Markers of active inflammation are raised ESR, C-reactive protein and immune complex levels. A major complication of systemic vasculitis is renal failure due to glomerulonephritis which can be detected by raised serum creatinine and urea.

(d) Specific markers of disease include anti-neutrophilic cytoplasm antibody (ANCA) in Wegener's, HLA-B27 in seronegative arthropathy and double-stranded DNA antibody in SLE.

(e) A chest X-ray may detect bilateral hilar lymphadenopathy in sarcoidosis and pleural effusion in SLE.

Management

These patients require immediate immunosuppression to prevent irreversible ischaemic damage to the retina and optic nerve head. Most will respond to high-dose systemic steroids or steroid-sparing agents such as cyclophosphamide, azathioprine or colchicine.

Prognosis

There is a high incidence of relapse following cessation of immunosuppression. Renal and cardiac involvement is common in these patients.

HIV microvasculopathy

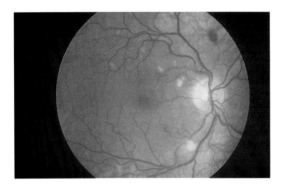

There are six cotton-wool spots in the posterior pole and peripapillary region in an otherwise normal fundus. This is consistent with HIV microvasculopathy which is the commonest posterior segment disorder found in patients with HIV. Other ocular problems associated with HIV include:[1]

- Anterior segment problems such as keratoconjunctivitis sicca, blepharitis, drug allergy, infective keratitis (such as herpes simplex or fungal infection), Kaposi's sarcoma, herpes zoster ophthalmicus and uveitis.
- Posterior segment problems such as vasculitis and chorioretinitis (due to cytomegalovirus or toxoplasmosis).
- Neuro-ophthalmological problems such as optic neuropathy, demyelination, neurosyphilis, cryptococcal meningitis and papilloedema.

Investigations

(a) Risk factors of contracting HIV include a history of intravenous drug abuse, blood transfusion and homosexual sexual practice.
(b) Full blood count, lymphocyte count (especially the CD4 subtype) and HIV testing should be performed.
(c) There should be a full ocular and systemic examination to exclude other organ involvement, such as pneumonitis and colitis.

Management

Although HIV microvasculopathy requires no treatment, the patient should be warned of the risk of other ocular complications listed above. The patient should be managed with a general physician with an interest in such patients.

Prognosis

HIV microvasculopathy tends to wax and wane, but rarely results in retinal ischaemia.

Reference

1.   Jabs, D.A., Green, W.R., Fox, R. *et al.* (1989) Ocular manifestations of acquired immune deficiency syndrome. *Ophthalmology*, **96**, 1092–9

Acute posterior multifocal placoid pigment epitheliopathy (APMPPE)

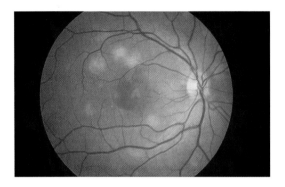

There are multiple well-circumscribed flat greyish lesions involving the retinal pigment epithelium at the posterior pole with normal overlying retina. With a history of a flu-like illness prior to the onset of visual symptoms, this is suggestive of acute posterior multifocal placoid pigment epitheliopathy (APMPPE), a bilateral lesion which affects young adults between the ages of 20 and 40 years. The central vision is usually affected but usually recovers with time. Other signs include perivasculitis, papillitis, iridocyclitis and tortuosity of retinal veins. It is also associated with erythema nodosum, episcleritis and hearing loss.

Differential diagnosis

Includes serpiginous (geographic) choroiditis (although this is usually found in an older age group with the lesions found in a peripapillary region and unilateral), presumed ocular histoplasmosis syndrome and multiple evanescent white dot syndrome.

Investigations

- The majority of patients complain of a preceding viral-like illness such as upper respiratory tract infection.
- Fluorescein angiography (FFA) reveals absence of fluorescence in the areas of active disease in the early prearterial phase of the angiogram with characteristic staining of the lesions in the late (after 30 minutes) phase. When the lesions have healed, there is retinal pigment epithelium atrophy with pigment clumping which shows up on FFA as areas of 'window-defects'.

Management

1.   As the majority of the lesions resolve spontaneously, there is no need for intervention.
2.   No treatment is required unless SRNVM develops.

Prognosis

Although visual recovery may take several months, the majority of patients achieve a final vision of 6/9. There may be a residual paracentral scotoma and a rare complication of subretinal neovascular membrane formation (SRNVM). Recurrences are rare.

New vessels elsewhere

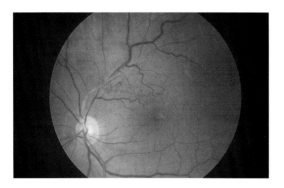

There is sprouting of fine blood vessels in a radial pattern from a periph-eral arteriole and is suggestive of neovascularization in the peripheral retina or new vessels elsewhere (NVE). Although there is no leakage of hard exudates, there are cotton-wool spots and blot haemorrhages adjacent to the NVE. This is associated with disorders which cause retinal ischaemia such as proliferative diabetic retinopathy, ischaemic branch vein occlusion, sickle-cell anaemia, longstanding retinal detachment, retinopa-thy of prematurity, leukaemia, Eale's disease and familial exudative vitreoretinopathy (Criswick–Schepens syndrome).

Investigations

(a) A full blood count, blood viscosity and fasting glucose level may help with the diagnosis of systemic haematological disorders (such as leukaemia) and diabetes.

(b) Careful fundal examination of the diseased and fellow eye will exclude other forms of neovascularization such as rubeosis irides and new vessels at the disc (NVD).

(c) Fluorescein angiography identifies the NVEs which manifests as discrete areas of dye leakage. It also identifies ischaemic retina which shows up as areas of non-perfusion.

Management

1. Treat the underlying systemic disease such as diabetes or leukaemia.

2. Single areas of NVE are amenable to sectoral argon laser photoco-agulation and often regress within 2–3 weeks of treatment. Repeat treatment will be necessary if there is no improvement. However, if there is more than two quadrants of ischaemia, panretinal photoco-agulation may be required to prevent further neovascularization.

Optic disc

Case 6.1

Optic disc drusen

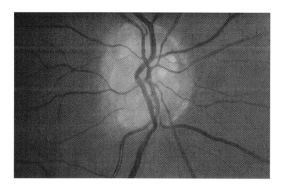

There is waxy pearl-like material in the optic disc, within the optic nerve head. This is consistent with optic disc drusen and is bilateral in 75% of cases. They are found in 0.3% of the population (there is a dominant inheritance pattern) and are associated with retinitis pigmentosa and angioid streaks found in pseudoxanthoma elasticum.[1] There is, however, no correlation between these drusen and drusen in the macula.

The majority of these cases are incidental findings and asymptomatic. However, they may cause visual problems by causing field defects, peripapillary haemorrhages or SRNVM.

Differential diagnosis

The differential diagnosis is a true optic disc swelling of any cause such as papilloedema and papillitis. Unlike papilloedema, the optic discs with drusen have no physiological optic disc cupping, show anomalous retinal vasculature pattern such as trichomatous branching, have a healthy pink colour and have retinal veins which pulsate.

Investigations

(a) Binocular examination to confirm the lumpy disc appearance (although they may be deeper within the optic disc) in the patient and immediate relatives, and exclude associated complications.
(b) Visual field assessment may detect characteristic patterns of field defects which may be either an enlarged blind spot (when the drusen is deeply buried) or a neuro-bundle defect (when the drusen is more superficial).
(c) Ultrasound and CT scan may detect calcification within the drusen.
(d) Fluorescein angiography is unnecessary but will show autofluorescence and late staining of the drusen. In addition, the anomalous retinal vessel branching may be detected.

Management

1.   Nil for asymptomatic cases.
2.   The patient does not require follow-up but ensure that the patient is aware of possible complications.

Reference

1.   Tso, M.O. (1981) Pathology and pathogenesis of drusen of the optic nerve head. *Ophthalmology*, **88**, 1066–80

Optic disc pit

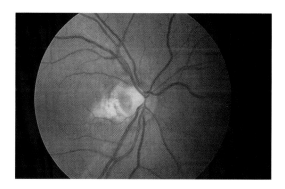

There is a round excavation located in the inferotemporal portion of the optic disc which appears darker than the surrounding disc tissue. This is consistent with an optic disc pit which is often unilateral. Complications may arise in 40% of these cases with the development of cystic changes in the macula which may progress into a macular hole or serous retinal detachment.[1]

Differential diagnosis

Differential diagnosis of an optic disc pit is an optic disc cupping from any cause.

Investigations

(a) Binocular examination of both eyes.
(b) Fluorescein angiography may reveal fluorescein leakage arising from the optic disc pit which fills up the area of serous detachment at the macular.

Management

There is no general agreement on the management, although the following options are possible.

1. Observe and do nothing. Some serous detachments reattach spontaneously.
2. Argon laser to the edge of the pit (thought to cause retinal pigment epithelium changes which may limit the spread of serous fluid).
3. Argon laser to the pit itself but with the risk of damage to the optic nerve head.
4. Vitrectomy and internal gas tamponade.

Prognosis

Poor in the presence of a serous retinal detachment of the macula.

Reference

1. Sobol, W.M., Blodi, C.F., Folk, J.C. *et al.* (1990) Long-term visual outcome in patients with optic nerve pit and serous retinal detachment of the macula. *Ophthalmology*, **97**, 1539–42

Optic neuritis

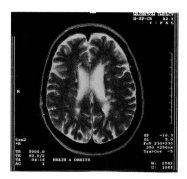

There are multiple bright lesions around the periventricular area in the CT scan of the brain suggestive of demyelinating plaque. This is consistent with a demyelinating disease such as multiple sclerosis, which is often unilateral. Other causes include:

- Idiopathic.
- Post-viral (infectious mononucleosis, herpes zoster) infection.
- Granulomatous infections, such as tuberculosis, syphilis and sarcoidosis.
- Orbital inflammation around the optic nerve (tuberculosis, syphilis).

The commonest cause of visual disturbance in demyelinating disease is optic neuritis which manifests as a retrobulbar neuritis, optic papillitis or, rarely, Leber's idiopathic stellate maculopathy (neuroretinitis). The ocular signs include:

- Decreased visual acuity and colour impairment.
- Central scotoma.
- Relative afferent pupillary defect.
- Motility problems such as internuclear ophthalmoplegia, gaze palsy secondary to nerve palsies and nystagmus.
- Uhthoff's phenomenon (worsening of symptoms from heat).
- Pulfrich's phenomenon.
- Swollen disc appears only with optic papillitis and neuroretinitis. The optic disc looks normal in retrobulbar neuritis.

Investigations

(a) Systemic examination to exclude other signs of demyelination.
(b) Visual evoked potentials (VEP) is delayed in 30% of cases.
(c) Visual fields.

(d)   MRI can detect demyelination plaques in the brain and exclude intracranial lesions which may affect the optic nerve and mimic optic neuritis.

Management

1.   Exclude other causes of optic neuritis.
2.   Optic neuritis secondary to demyelination usually resolves and requires no treatment. Corticosteroids given either systemically or as a retrobulbar injection have been tried but appear to have no effect on the final visual outcome. None the less, it appears to reduce the recovery period and is recommended in severe bilateral cases.

Prognosis

Although the visual loss may progress to its worst at around 2 weeks after the initial attack, 90% of patients will recover to near normal visual acuity, usually within 1–2 months. Younger patients have a better visual prognosis.

Papilloedema secondary to BIH

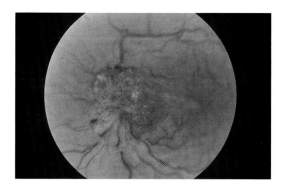

There is disc nerve fibre swelling with hyperaemia, peripapillary haemorrhages and cotton-wool spots with no loss of the physiological cup. This is consistent with benign intracranial hypertension (BIH) which is found mainly in women (8:1) under the age of 45 years. It is associated with obesity, endocrine changes (such as pregnancy, menstrual abnormality), drugs (OCP, steroids, antibiotics) and metabolic disorders (hypoparathyroidism, hyperthyroidism). At late stages, it loses the cup and has a 'champagne cork' appearance and finally pale atrophy.

Differential diagnosis

The differential diagnosis of optic disc swelling includes:

- Pseudo swelling (congenital 'full' disc, disc drusen, myelinated nerve fibres and hypermetropic disc).
- True swelling (papilloedema, papillitis, vascular causes such as CRVO and malignant hypertension, optic nerve compression, hypotony, toxic optic neuropathy and Leber's optic neuropathy).

Causes of papilloedema (swelling of the optic nerve produced by raised intracranial pressure) are:

- Intracranial space-occupying lesion.
- Benign intracranial hypertension.
- Carbon dioxide retention or lead poisoning.
- Guillain–Barré syndrome.

Investigations

(a) Systemic history will highlight raised intracranial pressure which manifests with symptoms of early morning headaches which are worse with coughing or bending down, visual obscurations, convulsions, nausea and vomiting.

(b)   Other ocular signs include VIth nerve ('false localizing sign') and IIIrd nerve palsies, afferent pupillary defects and fields defects.
(c)   CT or MRI scan will detect any intracranial space-occupying lesion and its compressive effects on the ventricles. However, in the case of BIH, the scans will be normal or show smaller than normal ventricles.
(d)   Lumbar puncture and CSF pressure measurement if BIH is suspected in the presence of a normal scan.

Management

1.   Treat underlying causes (weight loss, treat systemic conditions).
2.   Medical (diuretics).
3.   Surgery is indicated when there is evidence of visual field loss or afferent field defect. This may involve:
   • Repeated lumbar punctures.
   • Optic nerve fenestration improves visual function in 70% of cases.[1]
   • Neurosurgical shunting procedures.

Reference

1.   Sergott, R.C., Savino, P.J., and Bosley, T.M. (1988) Modified optic nerve decompression for pseudotumour cerebri. *Archives of Ophthalmology*, **106**, 1384–90

Opticociliary shunts vessels

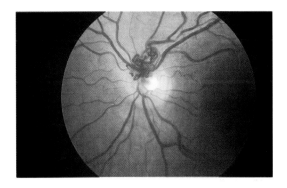

There are dilated venous loops present at the disc which look like optico-ciliary shunt vessels. This is consistent with a retro-orbital tumour such as an optic nerve meningioma. It typically affects women between the ages of 40 and 60 years of age and causes symptoms such as visual obscuration or visual loss when the optic nerve is compressed.

Differential diagnosis

Includes vessels which develop following central retinal vein occlusion, optic nerve glioma and craniosynostosis.

Investigations

(a) A careful history will exclude a previous episode of central retinal vein occlusion.

(b) A retro-orbital tumour may give rise to other signs due to optic nerve compression (such as decreased visual acuity, field defects, classically the junctional scotoma of meningioma, relative afferent pupillary defect, impaired colour perception), proptosis, choroidal folds and disc swelling.

(c) These vessels do not look like new vessels at the disc (NVD) as they form loops and are not thin and wispy. Fluorescein angiography can confirm the absence of leakage in shunt vessels.

d) A CT scan will localize the tumour and differentiate between a glioma (which arises within the nerve and forms an 'S'-shape) and a meningioma. The extent of the tumour can be appreciated to allow planning for surgery.

Management

1. A slow-growing tumour which is not causing any visual disturbance in an elderly patient (who may not want surgery) may only require regular observation.

2.   If there is visual loss, surgery is required to remove the lesion.

Prognosis

Surgery to remove and debulk the tumour is often successful with a small risk of tumour recurrence (very slow rate of growth). Optic nerve meningiomas in children and young adults behave more aggressively.

Optic disc hamartoma

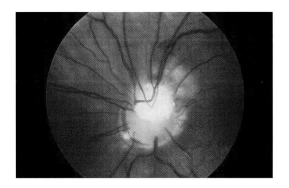

There is a solitary well-circumscribed and elevated lesion arising from the optic nerve head. This is suggestive of an optic disc astrocytic hamartoma which can be idiopathic or associated with a systemic disease such as tuberous sclerosis (Bourneville's disease) and neurofibromatosis (von Recklinghausen's disease). The lesion is initially translucent but later becomes white in colour and mulberry-like in shape and may be calcified. Complications are rare but progressive enlargement and subretinal exudation may occur.

Investigations

(a) An accurate history and systemic examination may reveal an associated dominantly inherited disorder such as neurofibromatosis and tuberous sclerosis. Other signs include adenoma sebaceum on the face and subungual fibromas.

(b) Calcification may be detected within these lesions using ultrasound or CT scan.

(c) Fluorescein angiography reveals a capillary network within the lesion.

Management

1. As the lesion is benign, treatment is not required.
2. However, associated systemic phacomases should be excluded as there are genetic implications to the patient's offspring.

Strabismus

Duane retraction syndrome

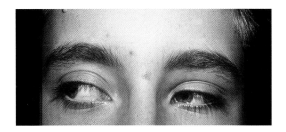

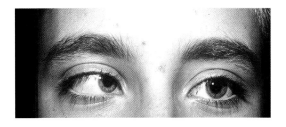

Duane syndrome is characterized by limitation of abduction, narrowing of palpebral fissure with globe retraction on adduction and a face turn to the affected side. Although mainly unilateral, 20% of cases are bilateral. The left eye is more commonly involved. Patients are rarely symptomatic and present either with a head turn or intermittent diplopia when it occurs in adults. Other signs associated with Duane's are anisometropia, amblyopia (20%), coloboma, heterochromia and microphthalmos. It is also seen in systemic diseases such as Goldenhar syndrome, Klippel Feil syndrome and cleft palate.

Differential diagnosis

Huber's classification divides the syndrome into three categories depending on the limitation of horizontal eye movements:

- Type 1 – Limited/absent abduction.
- Type 2 – Limited adduction.
- Type 3 – Limitation of both adduction and abduction.

Investigations

(a) Full orthoptic and extraocular movement assessment.
(b) Hess chart.

Management

1. Do nothing unless the patient is symptomatic.
2. Surgery is only indicated in the presence of:

- Manifest strabismus in primary position.
- Abnormal head posture, which is cosmetically unacceptable.
- Cosmetically unacceptable palpebral narrowing or ocular up/downshoots on adduction.

3.   Surgical options:
   - Recession (preferably on adjustable sutures) of the medial rectus of the affected eye to place the eye in a more central position and enlarge the field of binocular single vision is the best option. Avoid lateral rectus recession as this may lead to restrictive problems such as upshoot of the eye.
   - Lateral rectus muscle bifurcation and stabilization of one half above and the other below its original insertion can prevent slippage of the muscle over the globe.

Third nerve palsy

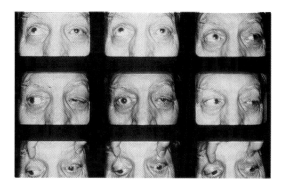

This is consistent with a left IIIrd nerve palsy which may be due to trauma, tumour, aneurysm (most likely to be a posterior communicating artery), diabetes or meningitis. Features that can be seen include:

- Ptosis.
- Exotropia on cover test (intorted and hypotropic).
- Absent EOM except abduction and intorsion. However, there may be muscle sequelae with overacting contralateral synergists (LR, SR, IR, SO) and contracture of ipsilateral antagonists (SR+/-SO).
- Test IVth by asking patient to look down and in, and watch for intorsion.
- Proptosis (lack of extraocular muscles tone).
- Enophthalmos (contraction at certain gazes).
- Pupil non-sparing and sparing.
- Aberrant regeneration, which can occur within 6 weeks in compressive IIIrd nerve palsy (pseudo-Von Graefe, lid-gaze dyskinesis, adduction on elevation +/-depression, enophthalmos on vertical gaze, IR innervation by MR fibres, abnormalities of pupil and accommodation).

Management

Management is tailored to individual patient requirements and depends on the extent of palsy (i.e. partial or complete), and when the patient presents. In early presentation it is usual to wait for 1 year to assess recovery of the nerve function. In late presentation the treatment depends on the amount of functional recovery. With a complete IIIrd nerve palsy where there is no possible recovery expected, the choices are to do nothing or to use an occlusive contact lens to prevent diplopia. In a partial nerve palsy with some recovery of function, surgery may be used to weaken overacting muscles to increase binocular gaze single vision (BSV).

Types of surgery
1.   Horizontal muscle surgery on affected eye. This involves either contralateral LR recession or a traction suture on MR in the affected eye to prevent LR contracture.
2.   Ptosis surgery. Brow suspension using Mersilene mesh or 4-O prolene sutures. Contralateral LR recession may be used in an eye with aberrant regeneration as it encourages adduction.

Sixth nerve palsy

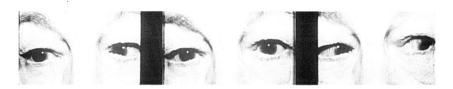

This is consistent with a right lateral rectus palsy whose aetiological causes are vascular (hypertension, diabetes, arteritides), tumour (false localizing sign) or inflammatory (sarcoid, meningitis). Other features which can be seen are

- Esotropia on cover-test (greater for distance).
- AHP (face turn to affected side).
- Muscle sequelae which consists of overaction contralateral synergist (MR), contracture ipsilateral antagonist (MR) and secondary inhibition contralateral antagonist (LR).

Investigations

(a) Exclude and treat systemic causes.
(b) Full orthoptic assessment.

Management

In the early stages one should wait for the natural recovery of the LR and prevent muscle contracture of the ipsilateral antagonist. If recovery does not occur, surgery is performed to keep the eyes straight in primary position and expand binocular single vision.

(1) *Early* The choice consists of either botulinum toxin to ipsilateral MR to prevent secondary contracture or prisms to prevent diplopia.

(2) *Late* (3–6 months later) This depends on the amount of functional recovery. If recovery is complete, the patient can be discharged. However if there is some recovery, the lateral rectus can be split in Jensen's procedure which harnesses the power from the superior and inferior recti, or transposed to the vertical muscles (Hummelsteim's procedure) thus increasing the range of abduction. Repeat botulinum injection to the ipsilateral MR may also be given as an adjunct.[1] However, if there is esotropia remaining, the contralateral MR can be recessed to prevent overaction of this yoke muscle. The ipsilateral MR should not be operated within 6 months of transposition surgery for fear of anterior segment ischaemia.

Reference

1.   Fitzsimons, R., Lee, J.P. and Elston, J. (1988) Treatment of sixth nerve palsy
     in adults with combined botulinum toxin chemodenervation and surgery.
     Ophthalmology, **95**, 1535–42.

Infantile esotropia

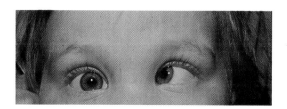

There is a manifest convergent strabismus in this child which is apparent on cover–uncover test. In the absence on any ocular abnormality and full extraocular movement, this is suggestive of either:

- Refractive esotropia which can be accommodative (due to hypermetropia) or non-accommodative (due to a high AC/A ratio).
- Infantile esotropia.

Differential diagnosis

Includes nystagmus block syndrome, VIth nerve palsy, divergence insufficiency or secondary strabismus such as sensory deprived or consecutive strabismus following previous ocular muscle surgery.

Investigations

(a) Full prenatal, ocular and systemic history should be taken.
(b) Orthoptic assessment of the strabismus to measure the angle of strabismus, amount of stereopsis, convergence-accommodative ratio and extraocular movement.
(c) Cycloplegic refraction and best corrected visual acuity. This will detect the presence of amblyopia and accommodative esotropia.
(d) Ocular and fundal examination to exclude abnormalities which may compromise the vision and result in a sensory deprived strabismus.

Management of the more common esotropias

1. Accommodative esotropia is due to the accommodative effort used in hypermetropia. In fully accommodative esotropia, spectacle correction is sufficient to correct the strabismus fully while partially accommodative strabismus will require surgery in addition to spectacles. The child should be followed up and refracted regularly to detect changes in the refraction as the degree of hypermetropia may decrease with age.
2. In non-accommodative strabismus with a high AC/A ratio, the strabismus can be corrected by reducing the accommodative effort

by using topical miotics and bifocal spectacles with a reading addition. In addition, surgery on the medial rectus muscles (either bimedial recession or Fadenisation) can reduce the AC/A ratio.

3.   Non-refractive infantile esotropia requires surgery to the ocular muscles to straighten the eyes. This involves recession of the medial recti and resection of the lateral recti (usually on the strabismic eye although either eye can be operated on). If there is a large coexisting inferior oblique overaction, an inferior oblique Z-plasty or recession can be performed in addition.

The child may have amblyopia secondary to the esotropia and will require occlusion therapy from the moment of diagnosis. Various methods of occlusion are available, including fogging with contact lens or spectacles or a topical cycloplegic, but patching is most commonly used. The duration of patching varies with the density of the amblyopia (the denser the amblyopia, the longer the duration). The child should be examined regularly to assess visual improvement and to watch for 'reverse amblyopia' whereby the vision in the good eye deteriorates from being occluded too often.

Brown's syndrome

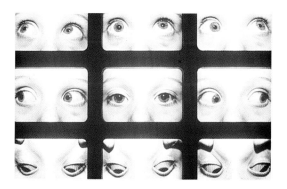

There is limitation of elevation of the right eye in adduction, and on right gaze the left eye dips below the midline. The rest of the extraocular movements are normal. This mechanical limitation of elevation in adduction is characteristic of superior oblique tendon sheath or Brown's syndrome. There may be an abnormal head posture, with the chin elevated and pointed to the opposite side.

Investigations

(a) There may be a history of head tilt and diplopia although this is usually absent in congenital cases. It is important to rule out secondary causes of Brown's syndrome such as trauma (classically road traffic accidents with trauma to the orbit), tendon cyst or inflammation associated with arthritis and post-ocular surgery (i.e. superior oblique tuck) for superior oblique palsy.

(b) Examination of the extraocular movements will elicit limitation of elevation in adduction. There may be a cyst on palpation in the area of the trochlear and an audible click caused by the cyst as it passes through the trochlear. Inferior oblique paresis (which is rare) should be excluded by feeling some form of restriction on forced duction test of the eye under anaesthesia.

Management

1. Most cases of Brown's syndrome are asymptomatic and therefore do not require intervention. The hypotropia is only obvious when the child attempts to look up. But when the child's height increases with age, he/she will spend less time looking up and as such the condition becomes less noticeable. Also there may be spontaneous resolution of the syndrome.

2. Surgery is indicated when there is a marked and cosmetically unacceptable chin elevation, hypotropia in primary position, marked

downshoot on adduction or diplopia. There are many options and they include superior oblique recession, tenotomy, the use of a silicone expander or merely freeing the fascia around the tendon. In cases of trauma, it is important to perform a duction test and examine for any foreign bodies and scarring. Steroid injection into the trochlear region may be beneficial in inflammatory causes of the restriction.

3.   Any amblyopia should be treated.

Prognosis

There may be risk of superior oblique palsy postoperatively.

Seventh nerve palsy

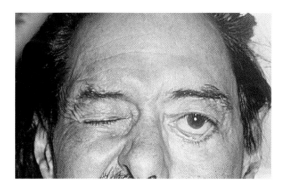

There is a failure of eye closure (orbicularis oculi muscle) and inability to smile on the right side. This is consistent with right VIIth nerve palsy. The distinction between upper and lower motor lesion lies in the ability to wrinkle the forehead; there is weakness of the lower face but normal forehead wrinkling in upper motor lesion due to bilateral representation at the brain stem nucleus from the cerebral cortex whereas all muscles are affected in lower motor lesions.

Causes of VIIth nerve palsy include:

- Intracranial lesions such as cerebrovascular accident, sarcoidosis, Bell's palsy, diabetes, hypertension and tumours such an acoustic neuroma affecting the cerebellopontine angle.
- Fracture of the base of the skull, otitis media, middle ear carcinoma or Ramsay–Hunt syndrome due to herpes zoster affecting the nerve as it passes through the temporal bone.
- Conditions affecting the nerve as it passes through the parotid gland such as facial trauma, surgery, tumour or inflammation (in sarcoidosis called uveo-parotid fever) of the parotid gland.

Investigations

(a) Exclude systemic causes such as tumours, sarcoidosis, diabetes etc.
(b) There are four aspects to the nerve that can be tested.
- Motor supply to the muscles of facial expression. Test frontalis muscle (ability to wrinkle forehead), orbicularis oculi muscle (the extent of eye closure, the amount of cornea show when complete closure is attempted, Bell's reflex, the amount of blinking and corneal wetting should be documented) and levator labii superioris and anguloris (ability to smile and show the teeth). The corneal sensation should also be tested as this affects management.
- Sensation to the anterior two-thirds of the tongue (relayed via the chorda tympani nerve).

- Secretomotor to the lacrimal gland (relayed via the greater super-ficial petrosal nerve).
- Stapedius reflex to noise is lost resulting in hyperacusis.

(c)   A headache with loss of hearing and corneal sensation should alert the clinician to a cerebellopontine angle tumour and would warrant either a CT or MRI scan.

Management

1.   All systemic diseases should be treated. Failure to find a cause suggests Bell's palsy as the aetiological factor.
2.   The eye should be protected if there is insufficient eye blinking and corneal exposure especially if there is poor corneal sensation. Temporary measures include lubricant ointment, eyelid taping, botulinum toxin-induced ptosis and temporary tarsorrhaphy as the nerve may recover over a period of time. Permanent palsy will require a permanent lateral tarsorrhaphy.

Jaw-winking (Marcus–Gunn) syndrome

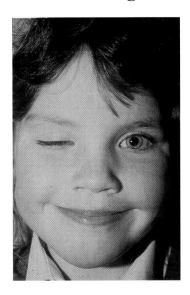 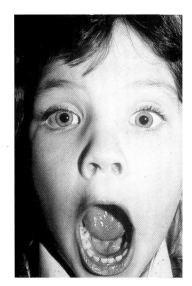

There is ptosis of the lid which is associated with retraction of the affected eyelid with opening of the mouth and jaw. This is consistent with the diagnosis of a jaw-winking or Marcus–Gunn syndrome which consists of eyelid retraction with stimulation of the ipsilateral medial pterygoid muscles. It is thought that a congenital connection exists between the mandibular portion of the trigeminal nerve and the oculomotor nerve supplying the levator muscle. It accounts for between 5 and 13% of congenital ptosis.

Differential diagnosis

Includes congenital ptosis and IIIrd nerve palsy.

Investigations

(a) The diagnosis is clinically obvious. However, it is important to exclude other causes of congenital ptosis such as a IIIrd nerve palsy.
(b) There should be a full orthoptic assessment as nearly 60% of these patients have some form of strabismus and amblyopia. A superior rectus weakness is often detected. In addition, the child should be refracted.

Management[1]

1. In the absence of ptosis-induced visual deprivation amblyopia, the condition can be left untreated as it may improve with age.

2. Amblyopia when present should be treated aggressively.
3. If there is strabismus (especially vertical strabismus), this should be treated before dealing with ptosis.
4. The eyelid surgical procedure depends on the amount of ptosis:
   - Mild ptosis and mild wink may require only a unilateral levator resection.
   - Moderate to severe ptosis requires unilateral levator excision of the affected side and unilateral or bilateral frontalis suspension using either autologous fascialata or Mersilene mesh.

Reference

1. Pratt, S.G., Beyer, C.K. and Johnson, C.C. (1984) The Marcus–Gunn phenomenon. *Ophthalmology*, **91**, 27–30

Orbit and oculoplastics

Thyroid eye disease

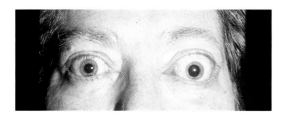

There is a wide-staring gaze with scleral show between the upper lids and cornea in both eyes. This is consistent with thyroid eye disease which occurs in 5% of thyroid patients. Eighty per cent have thyroid imbalance. TED precedes systemic disease by 18 months.

Investigations

(a) Thyroid hormonal status.
(b) Auto-immune profile.
(c) Colour contrast sensitivity.
(d) Serial Hess charts.
(e) CT or MRI scans.

In the majority of patients with thyroid disease, the eye is rarely affected and only requires observation. During follow-up, the patient should be monitored for:

- Optic nerve function.
- Proptosis.
- Ocular motility.
- Corneal exposure.

In the event of TED becoming active, orbital immunosuppression is required to prevent the build-up of GAG in the orbit causing ON compression, motility and cosmetic problems. Immunosuppression can be achieved using:

- Steroids (systemic, high dose for 6–8 weeks or pulsed i.v. 1 g methyl pred. for 3 days).
- Orbital radiotherapy 1500–2000 Rads in ten divided doses).
- Steroid sparing therapy (AZT 50 mg t.d.s. +/- low-dose steroids).

Azothioprine

Management[1]

There are four management levels in treating TED.

1. Orbital decompression either medically (using systemic steroids) or surgically when there is evidence of optic nerve compression.

2.   Strabismus surgery using adjustable recessions to enlarge BSV at the primary position when there is diplopia which has remained constant over the previous 6 months from the evidence of Hess charts.[2]
3.   Lid positioning for upper lid retraction that is cosmetically unacceptable.
     • Lowering upper lid with adjustable 5 or 6-O vicryol sutures.
     • Raising lower lid with lateral or medial canthal slings/scleral implant between LL retractors and tarsus/dividing LLR and place LL on traction/dividing LLR and recess to 15 mm behind limbus.
4.   Cosmetic surgery for 'puffy' eyelids (blepharoplasty, although patients are rarely satisfied).

References

1.   Fells, P. (1991) Management of dysthyroid eye disease. *British Journal of Ophthalmology*, **75**, 245–6
2.   Morris, R.J. and Luff, A.J. (1992) Adjustable sutures in squint surgery. *British Journal of Ophthalmology*, **76**, 560–2

Blow-out fracture

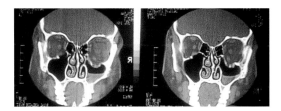

The CT scan demonstrates soft tissue herniation into the left maxillary sinus which has a fluid level. This is consequent to a direct blow to the orbit causing an increase in pressure within the orbit resulting in fracture of either the floor or the medial wall. Signs of a blow-out fracture include orbital emphysema, ecchymosis, hypotropia with high skin crease, limited ocular movement (especially vertical duction) and infraorbital nerve paraesthesia.

Blow-out fractures are divided into:

- Pure where the orbital rim is spared.
- Combined or 'impure' where the orbital rim is also fractured.

Investigations

(a) Skull X-ray (Water's view) to detect fracture, orbital emphysema, soft tissue herniation into the sinus ('pear-drop' sign) and fluid (blood) level in the maxillary sinus.
(b) CT scan.
(c) Serial Hess charts and field of binocular single vision.
(d) Proptosis/ecchymosis/enophthalmos.
(e) Visual acuity and colour vision.

Management[1]

Follow-up of the patient should be every 3–4 days for 2 weeks to assess the changes in ocular movements, proptosis and visual acuity. There are specific indications for early intervention otherwise blow-out fractures should be left.

1. *Early* (within 2 weeks) Orbital wall reconstruction to free prolapsed or incarcerated orbital tissue by placing a silastic plate over the fracture site if there is enophthalmos more than 3 mm, serial Hess charts which are not improving associated with persistent diplopia and significant soft tissue herniation into the sinus.
2. *Late* At this stage orbital fracture repair is usually less successful, the treatment is directed at any associated complications such as enophthalmos or diplopia. For enophthalmos Fascenella–Servat or

dermal fat graft to the superior orbital rim may disguise the cosmetic appearance. Surgery on extraocular muscles is only necessary if diplopia is persistent.

Reference

1.   Wesley, R.E. (1992) Current techniques for the repair of complex orbital fractures. *Ophathalmology*, **99**, 1766–72

Case 8.3

Dermoid cyst

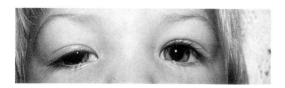

There is a smooth, round lesion in the superonasal aspect of the child. It should be cystic on palpation and not fixed. This is suggestive of a dermoid cyst which is a developmental choriostoma of ectoderm which is pinched off as bony suture lines close during development. Pathologically it is lined by keratinizing epithelium and contains embryonic epidermal derivatives such as hair, sebaceous gland and keratin. It presents either as an orbital lesion at the superotemporal-temporal aspect near the zygomaticofrontal suture (or less commonly superonasal) of the orbit or at the corneal-scleral junction. Although the majority arise *de novo*, some dermoids are associated with Goldenhar syndrome.

Complications arising from dermoid include:

* Cyst rupture or leakage of cyst content resulting in acute inflammatory response.
* Erosion backwards into the anterior cranial fossa and sinuses.
* Cyst infection.

Investigations

(a) X-ray may show characteristic indentation against the orbital wall or bony defects if the cyst extends intracranially.

(b) CT scan may outline any intracranial extension when planning for surgery.

Management[1]

1. Observation, as these cysts are slow-growing and often asymptomatic. It is important to ensure that the dermoid does not interfere with the child's vision and cause amblyopia.

2. Surgery to remove the cyst *en bloc*. Superficial orbital dermoids can be easily removed through a skin incision while deeper lesions may necessitate a lateral orbitotomy or even via a neurosurgical approach. It is important that total cyst removal is achieved to prevent a postoperative inflammatory reaction and recurrence.

Reference

1. Sherman, R., Rootman, J. and La Pointe, J. (1984) Orbital dermoids: clinical presentation and management. *British Journal of Ophthalmology*, **68**, 642–52

Nasolacrimal duct obstruction

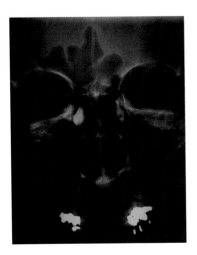

This is a dacryocystogram showing pooling of dye in the right nasolacrimal sac suggesting a complete blockage at the level of the nasolacrimal duct.

The causes of nasolacrimal duct obstruction are:

- Congenital (15% are non-patent at birth although the majority resolve by the age of 1 year).
- Acquired (ageing, trauma, chronic infection and previous dacryocystitis).

Investigations

(a) Examination of the punctum (exclude canaliculitis secondary to Actinomyces or herpes simplex), lid (exclude ectropion, trichiasis, blepharitis), marginal tear strip and corneal pathology (erosion) which may result in epiphora.

(b) The medial canthal area should be examined for a mucocele or tumour which may block the flow of tears. Gentle pressure over this area may result in regurgitation of mucus, pus or debris.

(c) Dilatation of the punctum with a Nettleship dilator, probing and syringing of the nasolacrimal duct.

(d) Jones test
- Primary test: 2% fluorescein applied on the conjunctival sac and 5 minutes later a white cotton bud placed by the nostril to check for flow through of the dye. In a positive test, there is recovery of the dye implying normal lacrimal duct.

- Secondary (irrigation) test: (residual fluorescein is washed out from the conjunctival sac and the nasolacrimal duct is irrigated with clear normal saline through a cannula inserted through the punctum. In a positive test, some dye will be recovered from the nose suggesting *partial obstruction* to the nasolacrimal duct while failure of dye recovery suggests complete blockage or lacrimal pump failure.

(e)   Dacryocystogram.

(f)   Lacrimal scintillography.

(g)   Nasal cavity examination (as tumours arising from the nose and sinuses can block the passage of tears).

Management[1]

The indications for surgery and the type of surgery required are as listed below:

1.   Congenital obstruction occurs in around 2–5% of full-term infants but will have completely canalized within a year after birth especially with some encouragement with massage of the lacrimal sac. However, should symptoms persist, probing may be required to perforate the thin membrane within the duct.

2.   Adult obstruction requires a dacryocystorhinostomy (DCR). If the blockage is at a higher level at the point where the common canaliculi enters the sac, then tubes may be required in addition. If the blockage is at the common canaliculi (but where there is more than 8 mm of canaliculi to allow anastomosis to the lacrimal sac), a canaliculo-DCR with tubes will be required. If there is insufficient patent canaliculi present, then a bypass Lester–Jones tube will be required to carry tears from the medial canthus into the nose.

Reference

1.   McNab, A. (1993). Lacrimal surgery. In: *Practical Ophthalmic Surgery*. (ed. H. Willshaw), Churchill Livingstone, Edinburgh, pp. 191–211

Involutional (senile) ptosis

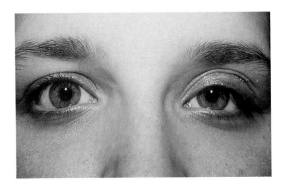

This is a ptosis in the ~~right~~ *Left* eye with a high skin crease and palpebral aperture of 4 mm compared to 9 mm in the fellow eye. This is consistent with involutional ptosis due to aponeurotic atrophy and dehiscence secondary to old age.

Differential diagnosis

1. Pseudoptosis. Patients with a microphthalmic or hypotropic (in double elevator palsy) eye and lid retraction in the contralateral eye may appear to have a ptosis.
2. True ptosis can be due to:
   - Mechanical (any lid tumour, dermatochalasis and oedema will cause a ptosis due to excess weight).
   - Neurogenic (IIIrd nerve palsy, Horner's syndrome or Marcus–Gunn jaw-winking syndrome).
   - Cicatricial (alkali burn, Steven–Johnson syndrome or pemphigoid).
   - Myogenic (dystonia myotonica, myasthenia gravis or chronic progressive external ophthalmoplegia).

Investigations

(a) The lid should be assessed and documented for amount of:
   - Ptosis.
   - Palpebral aperture.
   - Levator function (normal is between 15 and 18 mm).
   - Skin crease.
   - Lid position on downgaze (the lid lags behind in dystrophic conditions).
   - Fatiguability.

(b) Pupillary reaction tested to exclude IIIrd nerve palsy.

(c) Ocular motility tested to exclude IIIrd nerve palsy and aberrant regeneration.

(d) Fatiguabililty, Cogan twitch and hypometric saccades point to myasthenia.

(e) Bell's phenomenon.

Management

Management of a senile ptosis is to lift the ptotic lid to match the fellow eye preferably under local anaesthesia, to clear the lid off the visual axis, and ensure corneal exposure does not occur. The type of surgery depends on the amount of levator function:[1]

1. >10 mm with less than 2 mm ptosis (Fascanella–Servat procedure).
2. >10 mm with more than 2 mm ptosis (aponeurosis advancement).
3. 4–10 mm (levator resection).
4. <4 mm (brow suspension using either Mersilene mesh or fascialata).

Reference

1. Collin, J.R.O. (1989) *A Manual of Systemic Eyelid Surgery*, 2nd edn, Churchill Livingstone, Edinburgh, pp. 39–74

Basal cell carcinoma

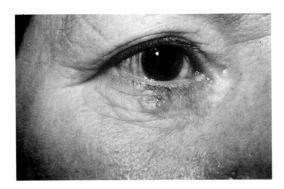

There is an elevated lesion measuring 1 cm in diameter arising from the lower lid and which appears to have an ulcerated centre and raised edges with telangiectasia. This is consistent with a basal cell carcinoma and is commonly found on the medial aspect of the lower lids of elderly patients with a history of ultraviolet light exposure or in xeroderma pigmentosa. There are two main forms of basal cell carcinoma (BCC), the nodular (which has well-defined rolled edges) and sclerosing or morpheaform (flat and spreads beneath normal epidermis).

Differential diagnosis

Includes a squamous cell carcinoma, Bowen's disease and Meibomian gland carcinoma.

Investigations

(a) History of a slow growth is suggestive of a BCC while more rapid expansion suggests the more sinister squamous cell carcinoma.
(b) A biopsy will confirm the diagnosis and help the planning of surgery.
(c) Examination should be carried out for other co-existing lesions, especially in xeroderma pigmentosa.

Management

The lesion should be excised as soon as possible to prevent further growth which may make lid reconstruction difficult.

1. *Cryotherapy* if the lesion is small or in multiple cases in xeroderma pigmentosa or BC naevus syndrome which is an autosomal dominant dermatosis associated with systemic abnormalities such as jaw cysts, congenital skeletal abnormalities and hand pits. There may be hundreds of these lesions which are best treated with cryotherapy as excessive surgery may be disfiguring.

2.   *Radiotherapy* only if the lesion is away from ocular structures due to the risk of dry eye.
3.   There are two aspects to surgery – excision and repair:[1,2]
     - Excision with a 3 mm margin is universally considered to be successful in removing tumour in total. Frozen sections using Moh's micrographic technique of checking the resection margins may ensure total removal.
     - Repair of the lesion may be difficult if the defect is large (i.e. more than half a lid). The options for a small defect (less than half a lid) are direct closure, especially if sufficient lid laxity is present. Otherwise, a lateral cantholysis or semicircular (Tenzel) flap of skin and orbicularis muscle may provide laxity to close the defect. A large defect (more than half a lid) requires either a free skin graft with tarso-conjunctival flap from the superior lid (Hughes procedure), or free tarsal graft with skin mobilization.

Prognosis

Excellent 5-year survival, as they do not metastasize. Even if there is residual tumour remaining, there is only a 5% risk of recurrence. Medial canthal BCC have a poorer prognosis as they can extend posteriorly into the sinuses.

References

1.   Collin, J.R.O. (1989) *A Manual of Systemic Eyelid Surgery*. 2nd edn, Churchill Livingstone, Edinburgh, pp. 76–95
2.   Older, J.J. (1987) *Eyelid Tumours: Clinical Diagnosis and Surgical Treatment*, Raven Press, New York, pp. 9–13

Post-enucleation socket syndrome (PESS)

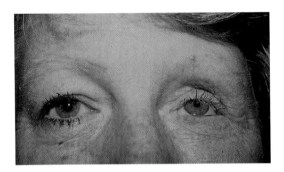

This is consistent with post-enucleation socket syndrome or PESS which is due to insufficient volume of the orbital replacement implant and downward and backward rotation of orbital contents resulting in a sunken look with a high skin crease and hypotropia (and enophthalmos) of the prosthesis. When the prosthesis is removed, the inferior fornix is likely to be absent. Other complications associated with enucleation include implant extrusion, superior sulcus deformity and blepharoptosis (due to a decrease in orbital volume), conjunctival shrinkage and eyelid laxity.

Management

The management is twofold. First, increase the orbital volume, using the following methods:

1. A secondary implant if no implant had been inserted following the enucleation.
2. Replacing the present implant with another implant of a larger volume.
3. Placement of dermis fat graft to the upper lid.[1]

Secondly, correct eyelid laxity:

4. The lower fornix needs to be deepened to support the prosthesis. This is achieved using fornix deepening sutures with a mucous membrane graft harvested either from buccal or nasal mucosa.
5. The high skin crease is not due to aponeurosis dehiscence but is caused by a smaller orbital volume. This can be solved by the placement of silicon or Teflon material in the subperiosteal space on the orbital floor to move the orbital contents forward to fill the superior sulcus.
6. Eye lid laxity requires a lateral canthal tendon sling to pull the lower lid laterally and tighten it. This is important as the lower lid plays a crucial part in keeping the prosthesis in the orbit.

Prognosis

It is thought that hydroxyapatite orbital implant following enucleation may reduce the extent of PESS due to the larger volume compared to a silicone.

Reference

1. Archer, K.F. and Hurwitz, J.J. (1989) Dermis-fat grafts and evisceration. *Ophthalmology*, **96**, 170–4

Herpes zoster ophthalmicus

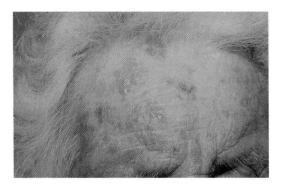

This is consistent with herpes zoster in the ophthalmic division of the trigeminal nerve due to reactivation of the latent virus in the trigeminal ganglion following the primary infection as chicken-pox at an earlier occasion. In over half these cases, there is ocular involvement especially when there is involvement of the external branch of the nasociliary nerve dermatome at the tip of the nose (Hutchinson's sign). The ocular features can be divided into:[1]

- Inflammatory changes such as conjunctivitis, episcleritis, keratoscleritis, nummular or dendritic keratitis, iridocyclitis, papillitis and retinal necrosis.
- Neurological changes such as neuropathic keratitis, ocular muscle palsy and post-herpetic neuralgia.
- Scar formation such as disciform keratitis, lipid keratopathy, scarring of the lid and skin.

Differential diagnosis

Includes zosterform herpes simplex and impetigo.

Investigations

Although the diagnosis is mainly a clinical one, culture of the vesicle fluid with immunofluorescent labelling will differentiate a viral from a bacterial cause.

Management

The aim of treatment is to limit viral replication as early as possible, limit scar formation and deal with late complications such as post-herpetic neuralgia and lid scarring.

1.	Systemic antiviral therapy with acyclovir appears to reduce the duration of the rash and the neuralgia when administered early in the vesicular stage of the disease. It can be given intravenously (at 10 mg/kg over an hour 3 times daily) or orally (at 800 mg 5 times daily).
2.	The skin rash can be treated with topical antiviral (idoxuridine or acyclovir) in the vesicular stage to reduce the viral load and appears to reduce the incidence of post-herpetic neuralgia. During the healing stage, topical anti-inflammatory steroid ointment or cream may be used to limit the extent of scar formation while antibiotic preparations can prevent secondary bacterial infection.
3.	Systemic steroid is only indicated if there is evidence of optic neuritis, cerebral angitis, large haemorrhagic skin bullae or total ophthalmoplegia.
4.	Pain control is essential during both the disease and post-herpetic period.
5.	Acute inflammatory ocular complications (such as iritis and keratitis) should be dealt with accordingly during the disease period while scar formation such as lid or corneal scarring can be dealt with at a later date.

Tips

1.	Look for sectoral iris atrophy (characteristic of herpes zoster) by transilluminating the eye, or scarring of the dermatome.
2.	Corneal sensation is often reduced.

Reference

1.	Marsh, R.J. and Cooper, M. (1992) Ophthalmic herpes zoster. *Eye*, **7**, 350–70

Capillary haemangioma

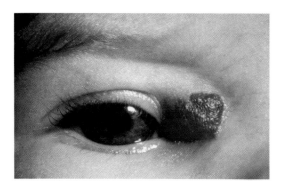

There is a red elevated cutaneous lesion on the upper nasal eyelid of this child. This is consistent with a capillary or strawberry haemangioma. It is often present at or shortly after birth, usually at the supranasal orbital region. The natural history is that it enlarges over the first 6 months and stays the same size thereafter. The majority of these masses undergo spontaneous reduction over the next few years, usually by the age of 7 years. There is a risk of amblyopia due to the visual occlusion by the mass causing a mechanical ptosis (visual deprivation amblyopia) or astigmatism (anisometropic amblyopia). Other complications include spontaneous haemorrhage and strabismus.

Investigations

(a) The diagnosis is a clinical one.
(b) Due to the risk of amblyopia, the child should be refracted and the vision should be assessed accurately to detect any reduction in vision due to visual deprivation.

Management

Due to the natural history of spontaneous resolution, no treatment may be required and the child seen on a regular basis to detect complications and to monitor the lesion. If the lesion is extremely large and causes a mechanical ptosis with a risk of amblyopia or if the parents are insistent on intervention, the following modalities of treatment may be offered.

1. Intralesional injection with steroids (such as triamcinolone or betamethasone) can reduce the tumour size in around 80% of cases.[1] Repeated injections may be required.
2. Low-dose radiotherapy may reduce the mass but has radiation side-effects.

3.   Surgical debulking has been tried but has the risk of bleeding and scarring of the skin.

Reference

1.   Kushner, B. (1982) Intralesional corticosteroid injection for infantile adenexal haemangioma. *American Journal of Ophthalmology*, **93**, 496–506

Cavernous haemangioma

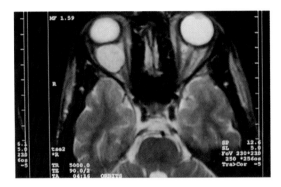

There is a large homogenous intraconal (within the muscle cone) lesion in the right orbit on CT scan. It is well-demarcated and encapsulated and is similar density to that of brain[1]. This is consistent with a cavernous haemangioma (a hamartoma) which presents between the ages of 30 and 70 years. It causes a slowly progressive painless proptosis. Visual disturbance may be due to metamorphopsia (arising from choroidal folds) or diplopia. Optic nerve compression is late due to slow growth.

Differential diagnosis

Includes optic nerve glioma, meningioma and metastasis.

Investigations

(a) B-scan ultrasound shows a sharp capsular border with high internal reflectivity.
(b) Angiography will demonstrate the 'flush' of the haemangioma.

Management[2]

1. Due to the slow growth of the lesion, it may be left untreated if there are no complications.
2. Surgery requires a lateral orbitotomy and removal of the lesion within its capsule *en bloc*. There is little risk of damage to neighbouring tissues as it is well-encapsulated and easily visualized.

Pathologically, it consists of wide endothelial lined, blood filled channels separated by fibrous trabeculae. The lesion is surrounded by a capsule.

Reference

1. Orcutt, J.C., Wulc, A.E., Mills, R.P. and Smith, C.H. (1991) Asymptomatic orbital cavernous haemangiomas. *Ophthalmology*, **98**, 1257–60
2. Shields, J.A., Shields, C.L. and Eagle, R.C. (1987) Cavernous haemangioma of the orbit. *Archives of Ophthalmology*, **109**, 853

Orbital cellulitis

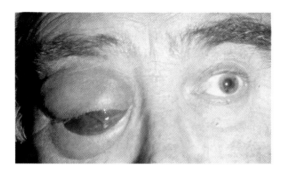

There is erythema, periorbital oedema, proptosis with conjunctival hyper-aemia and chemosis of the right eye. This is consistent with orbital celluli-tis which can be secondary to external eyelid infections (such as stye or laceration), dacryocystitis, retained foreign body and upper respiratory tract infection with sinus involvement. Organisms commonly involved include *Haemophilus influenzae* (in children), Staphylococcus and Streptococcus.

Cellulitis can be divided into preseptal (confined within the eyelid tissues) or orbital (within the orbit) cellulitis. The later is more ominous and is an ophthalmic emergency due to the associated complications such as orbital abscess formation, cavernous sinus thrombosis, brain abscesses and meningitis. In addition, the vision may be compromised due to pressure on the optic nerve and external ophthalmoplegia (where there is little extraocular movement due to tightness within the orbit) with increas-ing pressure within the orbit.

Investigations

(a) Ocular and systemic examination. Ocular examination should include measurement of visual acuity and colour perception, propto-sis, pupillary reflexes (to detect a relative afferent pupillary defect) and extraocular movements. Systemic examination should include an ear–nose–throat examination.

(b) An elevated white cell count may be seen on a full blood count.

(c) Blood and tissue cultures may be useful in identifying the offending organism.

(d) An orbital X-ray will exclude a retained radio-opaque foreign body.

(e) A CT scan or MRI scan will demonstrate the extent of orbital celluli-tis and any sinus involvement. It will also detect a brain abscess.

Management

This is both an ophthalmic and medical emergency and requires hospital admission and prompt treatment.

1. Systemic antibiotics (intravenous or oral) will be required to eradicate the infection.
2. Retained foreign body or abscess formation will require surgical drainage.
3. Surgical intervention is also required if the patient develops decreasing visual acuity or a relative afferent pupillary defect. Surgery in the form of orbital decompression will relieve the pressure on the optic nerve.

Blepharospasm

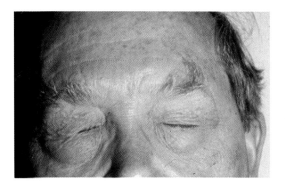

There is intense contracture of both eyelids suggestive of focal spasm of the orbicularis muscles due to essential blepharospasm. Other causes include Meige syndrome (where the spasm includes other muscles such as lower face and mouth, innervated by the VIIth cranial nerve) or hemifacial spasm. The symptoms experienced by the patient vary from mild irritation to spasm-induced visual disturbance which can prevent driving or reading. Blepharospasm usually occurs in females between the ages of 40 and 60 years.

Investigations

(a) An accurate history and careful observation during the muscle spasm will confirm the diagnosis.

(b) Exclude blepharospasm due to ocular irritative causes such as trichiasis, entropion, keratitis and keratoconjunctivitis sicca or a posterior fossa tumour.

(c) Symptoms such as headaches and visual obscurations which suggest an intracranial lesion warrant a CT or MRI scan.

Management

1. Medical treatment such as clonazepam, diazepam and haloperidol have been tried but with little benefit.

2. Acupuncture, counselling and biofeedback may offer benefit to some patients.

3. Botulinum-A toxin subcutaneous injection of 20 units to the orbicularis muscles provides a temporary paralysis of the muscles for 10–12 weeks. The toxin causes a presynaptic blockade of the neuromuscular junction and prevents the release of acetylcholine.[1]

4. Surgery involving selective avulsion of the facial nerve branches (Reynold's procedure) which innervates the orbicularis muscles can

be performed. Complications include delayed recurrences in 50% of patients, lagophthalmos and paralytic ectropion.

5.   Ophthalmic stripping. *Excision of eyelid protractors orbicularis (Andusons procedure)*

Reference

1.   Scott, A., Kennedy, R. and Stubbs, H. (1985) Botulinum-A toxin injection as a treatment for blepharospasm. *Archives of Ophthalmology*, **103**, 347–50

Carotid-cavernous fistula

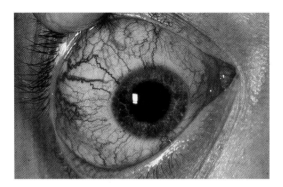

There is engorgement of dilated episcleral vessels with raised intraocular pressure in this eye following a history of trauma. This may be a sign of carotid-cavernous fistula which can either be a direct fistula (high flow and high pressure), where the defect is between the cavernous sinus and the intracavernous portion of the internal carotid artery (ICA), or an indirect fistula (low flow and low pressure) where the defect is between the meningial branches of the ICA and the cavernous sinus. It is often unilateral and is associated with trauma to the head or hypertension where spontaneous rupture may occur.

The signs vary with the type of fistula.

- Direct. The signs and symptoms are often dramatic due to the high pressure/flow of blood. There is chemosis, hyperaemia and proptosis due to venous engorgement. This can cause ophthalmoplegia, raised intraocular pressure, anterior and posterior segment ischaemia and thus affect vision. Auscultation of the eye may reveal a bruit.
- Indirect. The signs are subtle and there may only be the dilated vessels and raised intraocular pressure. It may progress gradually to proptosis and ophthalmoplegia.

Differential diagnosis

Differential diagnosis of engorged episcleral veins includes pseudotumour, cavernous haemangioma or acute dysthyroid eye disease.

Investigations

(a) There may be a history of trauma or hypertension. The speed of presentation may differentiate between the two types of fistula.
(b) Exclude other causes of engorged veins such as pseudotumour, cavernous haemangioma or acute dysthyroid eye disease.

(c)   Colour doppler may be useful to check the direction of blood flow.

(d)   Angiography is diagnostic and localizes the lesion for treatment.

Management[1]

The fistulas may close spontaneously, especially the indirect type. Indications for treatment include loss of vision, increasing volume of bruit and pain.

1.   The fistula can be embolized by the radiologist using a balloon catheter or steel coils.

2.   Surgical closure requires ligation of the carotid artery.

Reference

1.   Keltner, J.L., Satterfield, D., Dublin, A.B. and Lee, B.C.P. (1987) Dural and carotid cavernous sinus fistulas: diagnosis, management and complications. *Ophthalmology*, **94**, 1585–600.

Sturge–Weber syndrome

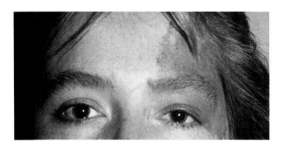

There is a cutaneous angioma involving the left ophthalmic distribution of the trigeminal nerve. This is consistent with encephalotrigeminal angiomatosis or Sturge–Weber syndrome, a phacomatosis with no inheritance pattern. Other systemic features include angiomas in the meninges and brain which can give rise to epilepsy and hypertrophy of the face on the affected side. Ocular features include secondary open angle glaucoma due to increased episcleral venous pressure, episcleral haemangioma and diffuse choroidal haemangioma in around 50% of patients.

Investigations

(a) The patient should be examined for associated ocular features, especially intraocular pressure.[1] Glaucoma may be bilateral in 10% of cases. Gonioscopy reveals an open angle and sometimes blood in the trabecular meshwork due to 'flush-back' from Schlem's canal.

(b) A CT scan should be performed in a patient with a history of epilepsy.

Management

1. In most cases, there is no need for any intervention.
2. However, in the presence of secondary open angle glaucoma, the intraocular pressure should be reduced to prevent field defects.

Reference

1. Iwach, A.G., Hoskins, H.D., Hetherington, J. and Shaffer, R.N. (1990) Analysis of surgical and medical management of glaucoma in Sturge-Weber syndrome. *Ophthalmology*, **97**, 904–9

Blepharitis

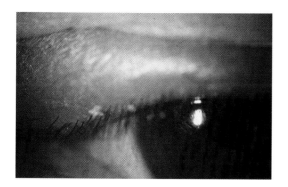

There are obvious crusts on the hair follicles and a cyst in the upper lid of this patient. This is consistent with a Meibomian cyst (also known as chalazion) secondary to blepharitis. Blepharitis and chalazions are associated with poor lid hygiene and skin disorders such as acne rosacea and ezcema, and are commonly found in children and elderly people.

Differential diagnosis

The differential diagnosis of recurrent blepharitis and chalazions includes a sebaceous cell carcinoma which carries a high (40%) mortality due to its predilection for early lymphatic spread.

Investigations

(a) There may be a history of poor hygiene or pre-existing acne rosacea or ezcema.
(b) Look for characteristic skin lesions such as rhinophyma and greasy skin.
(c) Evert the lid to exclude a sebaceous cell carcinoma. A biopsy may be required in suspicious circumstances.

Management

1. Treatment of blepharitis is by regular lid hygiene with cleaning of the lid and lashes using a cotton-bud soaked in either baby shampoo or weak bicarbonate of soda in warm water. A course of systemic antibiotics such as tetracycline or topical antibiotics may be required in acne rosacea to reduce the bacterial flora.
2. Chalazions can be easily removed by incision of the cyst from the tarsal side and curettage.
3. Sebaceous cell carcinoma requires surgical excision with at least 5 mm of normal tissue on all sides of the margin of the tumour. Some specialists recommend exenteration for lesions over 2 cm in length due to the likelihood of lymphatic invasion.

Index